ANKYLOSING SPONDYLITIS

Ankylosing Spondylitis

MICHAEL H. WEISMAN, MD

OXFORD
UNIVERSITY PRESS

OXFORD
UNIVERSITY PRESS

*Oxford University Press, Inc., publishes works that further Oxford University's
objective of excellence in research, scholarship, and education.*

Oxford   New York
Auckland   Cape Town   Dar es Salaam   Hong Kong   Karachi
Kuala Lumpur   Madrid   Melbourne   Mexico City   Nairobi
New Delhi   Shanghai   Taipei   Toronto

With offices in
Argentina   Austria   Brazil   Chile   Czech Republic   France   Greece
Guatemala   Hungary   Italy   Japan   Poland   Portugal   Singapore
South Korea   Switzerland   Thailand   Turkey   Ukraine   Vietnam

Library of Congress Cataloging-in-Publication Data

Weisman, Michael H.
Ankylosing spondylitis / Michael H. Weisman.
p. ; cm.
Includes bibliographical references and index.
ISBN 978-0-19-539910-3
1. Ankylosing spondylitis—Popular works. I. Title.
[DNLM: 1. Spondylitis, Ankylosing—Popular Works. WE 725]
RD771.A5W45 2011
616.7'3—dc22   2010041913

9 8 7 6 5 4 3 2 1
Printed in USA
on acid-free paper

CONTENTS

PART ONE INTRODUCTION AND OVERVIEW

1. Overview of Ankylosing Spondylitis 5
2. History of Ankylosing Spondylitis 11
3. Who Gets Ankylosing Spondylitis? 15
4. Anatomy of the Spinal Column 17

PART TWO WHERE AND HOW THE BODY CAN BE AFFECTED BY ANKYLOSING SPONDYLITIS

5. Clinical Presentation and Diagnosis
    of Ankylosing Spondylitis 27
6. Other Manifestations
    of Ankylosing Spondylitis 35
7. Bone Health 45

PART THREE ASSOCIATED CONDITIONS

8. Juvenile-Onset Ankylosing Spondylitis 51
9. Spondyloarthritis 57

PART FOUR DISEASE MANAGEMENT

10. Disease Management 71
11. Surgery 81
12. Physical and Daily Activity 87

PART FIVE THE FUTURE

13. What Does the Future Hold? 97
14. Frequently Asked Questions 103

Glossary 111
Index 119

ANKYLOSING SPONDYLITIS

PART ONE

INTRODUCTION

AND OVERVIEW

THE FIRST CHAPTER in this section, Chapter 1, provides a brief overview of ankylosing spondylitis (AS) and the criteria used by physicians to define AS. Detailed information about the disease process, its consequences, treatment, and management will be covered in later chapters. Chapter 2 presents an historical perspective, while Chapter 3 identifies who is most likely to have AS and why. Due to the fact that AS primarily targets the spinal column, the final chapter in this section, Chapter 4, reviews the anatomy of the spinal column.

1

Overview of Ankylosing Spondylitis

ANKYLOSING SPONDYLITIS (AS) is one of several conditions that belong to a group of chronic inflammatory rheumatic disorders known as *spondyloarthropathies* (SPAs). It is a chronic systemic inflammatory disease that primarily attacks the axial skeleton and adjacent structures. The axial skeleton (Figure 1.1) consists of 80 bones in the head and trunk of the body, and is divided into five parts: skull, ossicles of the inner ear, hyoid bone of the throat, rib cage, and the vertebral column.

Typically, the vertebrae of the spine become inflamed, causing chronic pain and discomfort. In more severe cases, this inflammation can lead to new bone formation on the spine, causing the spine to fuse in a fixed, immobile position resulting in a forward-stooped posture. If left untreated, the inflammation of the spinal joints will gradually destroy the cartilage and fibrous tissue of the surrounding structures as well as the ligaments and literally replace them with bone. There appears to be a cyclical process to the disease (Figure 1.2). Interrupting this cycle with early identification of the disease and aggressive treatment may prevent the immobility and stooped posture caused by spinal fusion.

The effects of AS are not confined to the spine. Patients with AS may experience pain and inflammation in other joints, such as hips, shoulders, knees, elbows, and feet. Ankylosing spondylitis may also affect the lungs, eyes, bowel

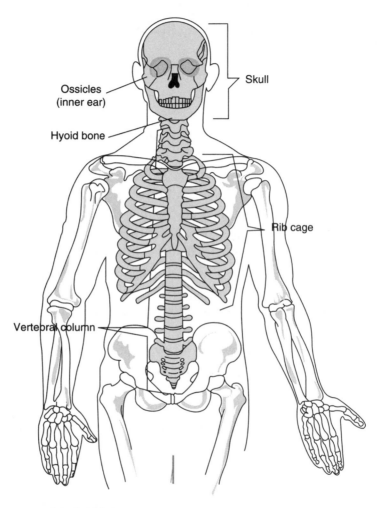

Ossicles
(inner ear)

Skull

Hyoid bone

Rib cage

Vertebral column

FIGURE 1.1 Axial Spine

and, in rare cases, the heart. There is a considerable genetic and clinical overlap between AS and inflammatory bowel disease, the causes of which are being investigated. Details of the effects of AS on other parts of the body, and the signs,

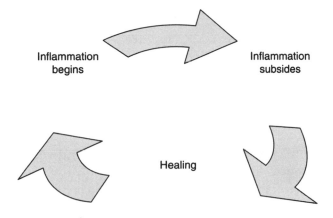

Inflammation begins

Inflammation subsides

Healing

FIGURE 1.2 AS Inflammatory Disease Process

symptoms, and treatment of conditions associated with AS will be discussed in later chapters.

CLASSIFICATION CRITERIA

The diagnosis of AS is based on clinical features and radiographic (X-ray) criteria. Unfortunately, there are no laboratory tests that can be used to establish a diagnosis of AS with certainty. The modified New York 1984 criteria (Table 1.1) are the most commonly used criteria to classify AS. Diagnostic criteria for AS have been recommended, but have not been validated through scientific study.

Classification criteria for AS, and other rheumatic diseases such as rheumatoid arthritis, are used to identify patients for research and genetic studies. To be useful for research, treatment protocols, and genetic studies, it is important that the classification criteria correctly and definitively identify patients with the disease. This means that the usual

Table 1.1

**MODIFIED NEW YORK CLASSIFICATION CRITERIA
FOR ANKYLOSING SPONDYLITIS**

Clinical Components

Low back pain and stiffness for ≥ 3 months that improves with
exercise but not with rest

Limitation of lumbar spine mobility in both the sagittal (sideways)
and frontal (forward and back) planes

Limitation in chest expansion as compared with normal range for
age and gender

Radiologic Component

Unilateral sacroiliitis of Grade 3 or 4, or bilateral sacroiliitis of
Grade ≥ 2

Diagnosis

Definite AS if the radiological criterion is associated with at least
one clinical component

Probable AS if:
- Only the three clinical components are present *or*
- Only the radiologic component is present

---

classification criteria identify patients with a disease that is
recognizable and quite certainly established with little doubt.
Because classification criteria almost always require changes
in the body that indicate that the disease has been present for
some time, it is difficult to develop diagnostic criteria ahead
of permanent damage. In the case of AS, classification criteria require X-ray evidence of damage to the spine. However,
we want to diagnose AS patients before spinal damage has

occurred; therefore, any diagnostic criteria need to be based on a probability that the patient has AS. This is the challenge that physicians face today in diagnosing AS—to develop diagnostic criteria that we can apply earlier in the course of disease and before damage has occurred to the spine. In other words, we want to diagnose patients with AS before or ahead of the time they fulfill classification criteria.

Fortunately, new classification criteria recently developed and refined by the Assessment of SpondyloArthritis international Society (ASAS) provide guidelines to aid in the diagnosis of patients prior to the appearance of positive radiographic findings.[1,2] The ASAS criteria use the presence of sacroiliitis (inflammation of the sacroiliac joints) by radiography or magnetic resonance imaging (MRI) with at least one feature of spondyloarthritis (SpA) or, the presence of HLA-B27 and at least two SpA as criteria for rheumatologists to use to assess the potential presence of AS prior to patients fulfilling the modified New York classification criteria. Although these classification criteria are new and have not yet been tested in the community in general, they do provide physicians with additional guidelines to make an earlier diagnosis before the disease has progressed to the point where X-ray changes have occurred. This is definitely a step in the right direction.

1. Rudwaleit M, Landewé R, van der Heijde D, et al. The development of Assessment of SpondyloArthritis international Society classification criteria for axial spondyloarthritis (part I): classification of paper patients by expert opinion including uncertainty appraisal. *Annals of Rheumatic Disease* 2009;68:770–776.
2. Rudwaleit M, van der Heijde D, Landewé R, et al. The development of Assessment of SpondyloArthritis international Society classification criteria for axial spondyloarthritis (part II): validation and final selection. *Annals of Rheumatic Disease* 2009;68:777–783.

2

History of Ankylosing Spondylitis

THE WORDS *ankylosing* and *spondylitis* are of Greek origin. *Angylos* means bent or crooked, and refers to the stooped or bent posture that may occur in AS patients. *Spondylos* means spinal vertebrae, and *itis* means inflammation. *Spondylitis*, then, is an inflammation of the vertebrae. The historical dating of ankylosing spondylitis (AS) is controversial and remains the subject of considerable debate, with some investigators dating the first incidence of AS to antiquity, while others contend that AS is of more recent origin. Based on paleopathologic studies—the study of diseases in ancient remains or medical writings—a number of researchers have concluded that evidence from humans and animals indicates that the origins of AS go as far back as several thousand years BC. For example, Egyptian pharaohs, including Amenhotep II (reign 1427–1401 BC), Ramses the Great (reign 1279–1213 BC), and Ramses' son Merneptah (reign 1213–1203 BC), have been described as having AS. During the fifth century, Hippocrates, author of the Hippocratic oath by which all physicians are bound to ethically practice medicine, described a condition suggestive of AS. Other researchers have determined that ancient cases of AS are more likely cases of a condition known as *diffuse idiopathic skeletal hyperostosis* (DISH), a calcification or a bony hardening of ligaments at the point of attachment to the spine. These researchers argue that paleopathologic studies are unreliable, and that only analysis with modern-day technology can definitively confirm the presence of AS. In partial support of their position, these researchers offer as evidence findings from a recent reexamination of the X-ray films of Ramses II; these films suggest that Ramses II did not have AS.

The skeletal remains of four generations of male members of the famous Florentine Medici family were studied to assess whether any of the four suffered from AS. After reviewing the remains of Cosimo il Veccho (1389–1464), his son Piero il Gottoso (1416–1469), his grandson Lorenzo il Magnifico (1449–1492) and his great-grandson Guiliano Duco de Nemours (1479–1516), researchers concluded that Cosimo and his son Piero had some type of spondylitis that may have been caused by AS or by Reiter's syndrome.

The first clinical description of AS was written by Bernard Connor, an Irish physician, in 1691 in his medical dissertation, although an earlier report by Realdo Colombo in 1559, describing what may have been AS, predates Connor's medical thesis. In his dissertation, Connor wrote that the vertebral bodies of the individual "were so straightly and intimately joined, their ligaments perfectly bony, and their articulations so effaced, that they really made but one uniform continuous bone."[1] (See Figure 2.1.)

Between 1691 and the first half of the nineteenth century, there were very few reports or clinical descriptions of spondyloarthritis (SpA) or AS. Clinical descriptions of AS became more frequent during the latter half of the nineteenth century. Sir Benjamin Brodie published a book, *Diseases of the Joints* (1850), in which he described the association between iritis, a complication of AS, and AS. A. Strumpell of Leipzig, Germany, Vladimir Bechterew of St. Petersburg, Russia, and Pierre Marie

---

1. Spencer DG, Sturrock RD, Buchanan WW. Ankylosing spondylitis: Yesterday and today. *Medical History*, 24:60–69, 1980.

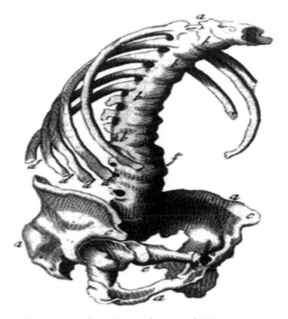

FIGURE 2.1 Fused Spine from Bernard Connor's Dissertation

of Paris, France, all neurologists, wrote three of the most detailed clinical descriptions of AS. The contributions of these three individuals were so significant that at one point, AS was known as *morbus Strumpell-Marie-Bechterew*. While each significantly contributed to our knowledge of AS, there are those that give primary credit to Pierre Marie for his description of both the anatomical and clinical features of AS, in findings he presented in 1898 to the Societe Medicale des Hopitaux de Paris. In 1890, an American, Bernard Sachs, joined the ranks of these esteemed Europeans when he published an account of AS as a "progressive ankylotic rigidity of the spine."

Most if not all of the early descriptions of the disease, of course, were made from autopsy studies. Technological innovations beginning in the late nineteenth century and continuing through the twentieth century allow for a more precise examination of the human body during life, and thus provide physicians with additional data with which to make a diagnosis of AS. One of the most noteworthy contributions was made by Wilhelm Roentgen, who discovered the X-ray, a diagnostic technique that enables physicians to take a picture of the spine and to observe changes in the spine as the disease progresses during a patient's lifetime. Another important diagnostic tool available to physicians is magnetic resonance imaging (MRI). MRI provides a detailed view of the internal structure of the body, and shows the contrast between different soft tissues in the body based on how these tissues line up in a magnetic field. An MRI can reveal inflammation of internal body structures, and this evidence of inflammation helps us make an earlier diagnosis of AS. This makes it a particularly useful diagnostic tool for use in patients with AS prior to those patients suffering from the bone changes that can be seen on X-rays.

What does the future hold for patients with AS? Although there is no cure for AS at the present time, the discovery of the association between the HLA-B27 antigen (see Chapter 3) and AS, as well as the discovery of new genes associated with AS, might provide a direction for targeted gene therapy and individualized treatment regimens. Further, these discoveries open the door to finding out how environmental triggers play a role in generating AS. After all, using the HLA-B27 antigen as an example, many more people have this gene but do not have AS. These discoveries might help us understand why only certain people with this genetic make-up get AS—what is it in the environment that triggers the disease and, ultimately, how can we prevent it?

Who Gets Ankylosing Spondylitis?

ANKYLOSING SPONDYLITIS (AS) is not a household word. Its consequences, however, are familiar to the estimated 2.4 million Americans who suffer from this devastating condition. Worldwide, AS affects between 1 in 100 and 1 in 200 adults. The prevalence of AS ranges from 0.3% to 1.5% in the United States, and varies by the ethnicity and the racial background of the population. AS is less common in African Americans, and it is frequently observed in some Native American tribes but not in others.

There is a strong genetic component to AS that varies by population in its frequency of occurrence. For example, the gene for AS is rare among the Japanese, and thus the disease is uncommon in Japan. However, in Finland and other Scandinavian countries, the gene occurs more frequently and AS is much more prevalent in these countries.

Men are more frequently affected by AS, although women and children are victims as well. The ratio of men to women with AS is 3:1; the reasons for male predominance are still unknown but currently under investigation. Ankylosing spondylitis usually occurs in young people between the ages of 16 and 35, with symptoms occurring rarely before the teen years. It is unusual for AS to develop after a person is 40 years old.

WHY?

Ah, the question, *Why AS?* The causes of AS have been under investigation for many years. A person's genes play a significant role and appear to be the most important factor, accounting for the lion's share of AS susceptibility. Medical researchers have known for years that there is a strong tendency for AS to occur in members of the same family, with most having the HLA-B27 gene. Two recently discovered genes, ARTS-1 and IL-23R, have been found to play a role in the development of AS. Four more genes have been discovered even more recently to be associated with AS—how these genes cause the disease to be expressed is under active study.

Researchers believe that environmental factors may influence not only the susceptibility but also the physical manifestations of the disease, as well as the timing of the appearance of the disease. Some scientists believe that a specific bacterial or viral infection may trigger the development of AS in people who are genetically predisposed. Because AS occurs so often in association with Crohn's Disease, it is felt that one route of environmental risk occurs through the gastrointestinal tract. This area is under very active investigation at the present time.

Anatomy of the Spinal Column

THE SPINAL column, also referred to as backbone, spine, or vertebral column, is one of the most important structures in the body. It houses and protects the spinal cord, provides structural support for the entire body, and gives us the flexibility and mobility that most us take for granted. The spinal column is a complicated structure that incorporates a combination of bones, joints, flexible ligaments and tendons, large muscles, blood vessels, and highly sensitive nerves. Because the inflammation associated with AS primarily attacks the spinal column, it is important to understand what the spinal column looks like and how it functions. Let's take a more detailed look at the structure and function of the spine, the workhorse of the body.

STRUCTURE AND FUNCTION OF THE SPINAL COLUMN

The spinal column is made up of the following parts:

- Back muscles
- Cervical spine
- Coccyx
- Curves of the spine
- Facet joints
- Intervertebral discs

- Lamina
- Ligaments
- Lumbar spine
- Pedicles
- Sacrum
- Spinal canal
- Spinal cord and nerve roots
- Thoracic spine
- Transverse and spinous processes
- Vertebrae

We begin life with a spinal column composed of 33 vertebrae, or bones. Over time, these vertebrae fuse, leaving the average person with a spinal column consisting of 24 vertebrae. Each vertebra is encased by a vertebral body that is cylindrical in shape, with an outside wall of hard cortex and an inside of soft marrow. The vertebrae of the spinal column are grouped into five regions, and the vertebral bodies increase in size from the top of the spinal column to the bottom. The regions, going from the top of the spine to the bottom, are the cervical vertebrae, thoracic vertebrae, lumbar vertebrae, sacrum, and coccyx (Figure 4.1). The cervical vertebrae are also referred to as the cervical spine. Similarly, the thoracic and lumbar vertebrae may be referred to as the thoracic or lumbar spine.

The first seven vertebrae, those that comprise the cervical vertebrae, are located at the top of the spinal column. The cervical vertebrae provide the flexible framework for the neck, as well as support for the head. These vertebrae allow us, for example, to nod "yes" or "no" and twist and turn our neck to give us the maximum ability to see and hear our environment. The next twelve vertebrae, the thoracic vertebrae, are the

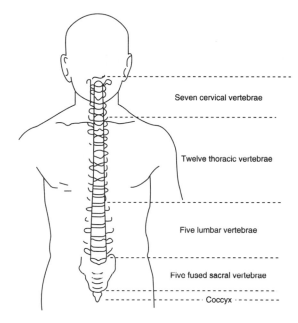

Seven cervical vertebrae

Twelve thoracic vertebrae

Five lumbar vertebrae

Five fused sacral vertebrae

Coccyx

FIGURE 4.1 Vertebrae of the Spinal Column—Front View

bones that form the rear anchor of the rib cage. The thoracic vertebrae form a transition between the cervical vertebrae above and the lumbar vertebrae below. The lumbar vertebrae, the five largest bones in the spinal column, are attached to many of our back muscles and function to support the body's weight. Below the lumbar vertebrae is the sacrum, a triangular shaped bone. When we are young, the sacrum has four or five vertebrae. Over time, usually by age 26, these sacral vertebrae fuse into a single bone. The sacrum is the back wall of the pelvic girdle. At the bottom of the spinal column is the coccyx, or tailbone. Like the sacrum, the coccyx begins with multiple bones (3 to 5) that become fused into one as we mature. In between each of the vertebrae that form the vertebral column are intervertebral discs. These discs are made of a fibrous cartilage core that acts as a shock absorber for the spine and our bodies, and allows the back to have flexibility by permitting the bones to have some freedom of movement.

When viewed from the side, the cervical, thoracic, lumbar, and sacral regions form corresponding curves called the cervical, thoracic, lumbar, and pelvic or sacral curve (Figure 4.2). The sacral curve is formed by the sacrum and the coccyx, the fifth spinal region. These curves are what allow us to stand upright; they also contribute to the maintenance of the balance of the upper body. It is interesting to note that the cervical and lumbar curves are not present in babies. The cervical curve forms when an infant begins to

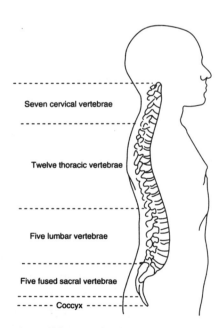

Seven cervical vertebrae

Twelve thoracic vertebrae

Five lumbar vertebrae

Five fused sacral vertebrae

Coccyx

FIGURE 4.2 Vertebrae of the Spinal Column—Side View

hold up its head, around the age of 3 months. The lumber curve develops as the child begins to walk. These curves are important parts of our balance and our stability. Obviously if there are exaggerated curves (such as in severe scoliosis) or there is no curve or it goes the wrong way (which might occur in late AS) the body becomes imbalanced, and pain and susceptibility to injury or damage may result.

Each vertebra in the spinal column has two sets of hinges called facet joints that join the back bones together and enable the body to move and bend. One pair of facet joints faces upward and the other set face downward (Figure 4.3). Facet joints are synovial joints. This means that the joint is enclosed by connective tissue and is nourished by a fluid that lubricates the joint, allowing it to move smoothly.

Threaded through the spinal column is the spinal cord, a large mass of nerve tissue that carries messages from the brain to other parts of the body, and from other parts the body to the brain. The spinal cord originates in the brain and leaves the brain through a hole in the base of the skull called the foramen magnum. When it leaves the foramen magnum,

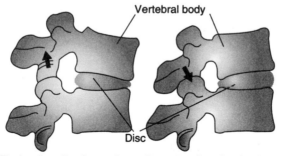

Vertebral body

Disc

Flexion (bending forward)   Extension (bending backward)

FIGURE 4.3 Facet Joints in Motion

the spinal cord winds through the spinal canal of the cervical, thoracic, and upper lumbar spine, and ends at either the first or second lumbar vertebrae. Nerve roots at the end of the spinal cord form a structure known as the *cauda equina*, or horse's tail. These nerves provide innervation to the lower trunk, legs, bowels, bladder, and sexual organs.

Surrounding the spinal cord is the spinal canal. The spinal canal includes the vertebral body, pedicles, lamina and, in the lower back region, the nerve roots of the lower spine. Like any building, the spinal canal is bounded at the lower and upper end by a floor and a roof. The floor is formed by vertebral bodies and the roof is formed by flat segments of bone called lamina. Pedicles reside on each vertebra and serve to attach the lamina to the vertebral body. On each lamina, there are two to three types of bony extensions, called processes (Figure 4.4). The spinous process is a bony protrusion that points straight back toward the skin behind the spine. You can feel these protrusions as bumps as you run your hands down your back. The transverse processes are a set of laminar extensions that vary in shape and form depending upon location in the spine. In contrast to the spinous process, which points back toward the skin, the transverse processes point out to the sides. Articular processes form the joints of the spine, attach the vertebrae to the joint surfaces and, like transverse processes, vary in form based on location in the spine. These joints allow us to twist, turn, and bend as we go about daily activities. Like joints anywhere else in the body, arthritis can occur in the spinal joints, causing pain and restricted range of motion.

The spinal column does not exist in isolation. Rather, it is supported by an intricate and complex group of muscles, ligaments, and tendons that help the spinal column function

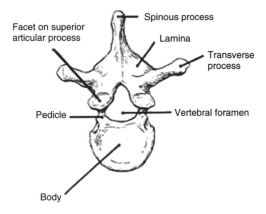

FIGURE 4.4 Articular, Spinous, and Transverse Processes

to support the body, hold it upright, and allow it to twist and bend. Muscle is a tissue made up of fibers that work to effect bodily movement. There are three types of back muscles that support the spinal column: extensor muscles, flexor muscles, and oblique muscles. The extensor muscles, responsible for helping hold up the spine, include the large muscles in the lower back and the gluteal muscles. The flexor muscles, as the names implies, allow us to flex, bend forward, and lift and arch the lower back. They are attached to the front of the spine and include the abdominal muscles. The oblique muscles allow us to rotate the spine and sit up straight, and are attached to the sides of the spine. Ligaments are composed of densely packed collagen fibers that connect bone to bone. In the spine, ligaments, like muscles, function to provide structural support and stability. Tendons are also made of collagen, and serve to attach muscle to bone. In a healthy individual, muscles, ligaments, and tendons in the back and spinal column work harmoniously.

PART TWO

WHERE AND HOW THE BODY

CAN BE AFFECTED BY

ANKYLOSING SPONDYLITIS

IN THIS PART OF THE BOOK, we review where and how the body may be affected by ankylosing spondylitis (AS). Chapter 5 details the effects of AS on the musculoskeletal system and reviews how a diagnosis of AS is reached. Chapter 6 continues with a discussion of the effects of AS on other affected organ systems: the eye, the heart, the lungs, the kidney, the genitourinary tract, the nervous system, and the gut. Chapter 7 deals with the bones, and the risk and prevention of fractures related to osteoporosis.

5

Clinical Presentation and Diagnosis of Ankylosing Spondylitis

ANKYLOSING SPONDYLITIS (AS) typically begins in young men between the ages of 15 and 25, and primarily attacks the musculoskeletal system—the muscles, bones, joints, and related structures of the body. In the early stages of AS, patients may experience fatigue, anorexia, and general physical discomfort. Because these symptoms are hard to pin down and can be associated with just about anything, AS is not suspected. In addition, patients without AS frequently complain of chronic back pain, and these two facts often result in a missed or delayed diagnosis, sometimes for many years. In order to try to understand how to make an earlier diagnosis and avoid these delays, we review how AS affects the musculoskeletal system, and the components of the medical evaluation required to diagnose AS.

CHRONIC INFLAMMATORY LOW BACK PAIN

Approximately three-quarters of AS patients experience some type of chronic inflammatory back pain. Scientists hypothesize that the cells involved in the inflammatory process release chemicals that stimulate the nerves surrounding the back bones, creating the sensation of pain. Initially, the pain is dull and intermittent. Over time, the pain becomes more persistent and will localize sometimes to the buttocks area or even in the small spinous processes that stick out of the back. It may also occur in the pelvis at the point where you sit down on a hard surface. One of the characteristics of this pain is that it tends to feel worse during periods of inactivity—at night in bed, for example, or after sitting in a chair for a prolonged period—with exercise or physical activity resulting in some pain relief. These features are what doctors refer to as "inflammatory back pain" and these may be used as clues to a diagnosis of AS. Typical characteristics of inflammatory back pain in patients with AS include:

- Younger age at onset of pain
- Pain and early morning stiffness of the spine or buttocks
- Improvement with exercise or other physical activity
- Gradual, insidious onset
- Symptom duration longer than 3 months
- Restriction of spinal mobility and deep breathing
- Difficulty sleeping due to pain
- Radiographic (X-ray) evidence of sacroiliitis or ankylosis
- Awakening at night because of back pain

Over time (usually measured in years), the progressive nature of AS can result in the flattening of the lumbar spine, leading to a loss of the normal inward curve (called the *lumbar lordosis*) of the lumbar spine and forming an exaggerated curve in the lower back in the other direction resulting in spine kyphosis, a condition more commonly known as a hunchback.

ENTHESITIS

Enthesitis (Figure 5.1) is an important feature of AS and may distinguish it from other diseases like rheumatoid arthritis. Enthesitis is characterized by inflammation at the sites of insertion of ligaments, tendons, or joint capsules to bone, and is the main cause of the pain, stiffness, and limited range of motion in the spine experienced by AS patients. Enthesitis often presents as swelling over the inflamed area, with patients reporting that the affected area is tender to the touch upon sitting or when touching selected objects. Sitting on hard surfaces can be extraordinarily difficult for a person with AS if the area covering pelvic bones is inflamed.

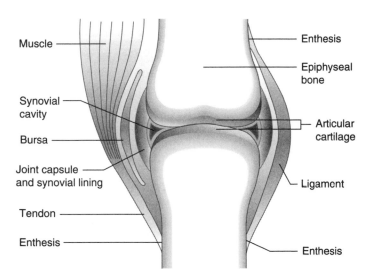

FIGURE 5.1 Enthesis

ARTHRITIS

Approximately one-third of AS patients will experience arthritis of the hips and shoulders, with the hip being particularly vulnerable. For reasons that are not completely understood, hip disease occurs frequently in adolescents during the earliest stages of AS. Exercises permitting movement of the hip and proper medical control may alleviate discomfort, increase mobility, and discourage rigidity from developing. Patients with AS also may experience peripheral joint synovitis, an inflammation of the synovial joints that occurs in about 50% of AS patients, targeting the hips, knees, ankles, fingers, and toes. This type of arthritis is very similar, but not identical, to the arthritis of a companion disease, rheumatoid arthritis. It appears to affect not only the synovial lining of the joints (as in rheumatoid arthritis) but it also affects the joint capsule, the enthesis attachments, and even the lining of the bones. The appearance of peripheral joint synovitis is different from rheumatoid arthritis in that it can affect an entire finger (not just the joints) or toe, and sometimes the locations can be just one, two, or three joints around the body in what seems like a random pattern.

OSTEOPOROSIS

Osteoporosis is another condition that frequently occurs in patients with AS. More than one-third of patients with AS may develop osteoporosis, a thinning of bone tissue and loss of bone density. Osteoporosis is related to disease activity and may occur very early in the course of AS, particularly when the disease is quite active. Osteoporosis places AS patients at an increased risk of vertebral fractures. Additional information about osteoporosis and the impact of AS on bones is provided in Chapter 7.

DIAGNOSIS

In Chapter 1, we mentioned that there are no definitive diagnostic criteria for AS. In the absence of diagnostic criteria, your doctor will rely on the results of your medical history, physical examination, blood work, and radiographic and other imaging examinations to diagnose the presence of AS.

A detailed medical history is necessary to determine your specific symptoms and whether you have a family history of AS. In order to obtain this information, your doctor will ask you a series of questions that should include: at what age did your back pain begin? How did your back pain begin—was the pain infrequent at the beginning, gradually becoming worse over time? Is the pain associated with morning stiffness that lasts for more than one hour? Does the pain improve with exercise or a hot shower? Does pain or stiffness in your legs or lower spine interrupt your sleep? Have your symptoms responded to over-the-counter medications such as Tylenol or Advil? Do you have any family members with AS? Because uveitis and inflammatory bowel disease are often associated with AS, your doctor should also ask whether you (or even a family member) have had these or other similar conditions.

After completing your medical history, your doctor will perform a physical examination to locate and pinpoint sites of inflammation. During the physical examination, your doctor will check for pain and tenderness along the back, pelvic bones, sacroiliac joints, chest, and heels. He/she should also check for any limitations in hip and spinal mobility, as well as restricted chest expansion. In addition to the physical examination, your doctor will also draw blood to test for the genetic marker HLA-B27, and for indications of inflammation. HLA-B27 is more prevalent, and is the primary susceptibility gene, in patients with AS. While it is found in up to 90% of AS patients, it is also found in about 7% of the general population depending on race or ethnicity. Simple blood tests for inflammation are an erythrocyte sedimentation rate (ESR) and a C-reactive protein (CRP). However, the presence or absence of HLA-B27, and raised ESR and CRP levels, are suggestive but not definitive for a diagnosis of AS.

The final component in the diagnostic evaluation is a radiologic examination. X-ray images of the sacroiliac joints are useful in determining the presence of bone damage. In the early stages of AS, though, there may be a lack of radiographic evidence. The presence of radiographic evidence means that the disease has progressed sufficiently to cause irreversible bone damage. In patients with a significant medical history, a physical examination positive for inflammatory sites and restricted range of motion, and insufficient radiographic evidence, physicians must rely on their clinical judgment to make a final determination as to the presence of AS. It is better for physicians to err on the side of inferring a diagnosis of AS before bone damage occurs so that treatment can be initiated as early as possible in the disease process in the hope of preventing future damage.

It has recently become possible to detect AS earlier in the disease process using magnetic resonance imaging (MRI). MRI is a noninvasive diagnostic imaging test that uses an electromagnetic process to allow for the visualization of the detailed internal structure of the body. MRI is sensitive to inflammation in soft tissues and bone, and can visualize these changes even when the X-ray is normal. It does not use external radiation, so it is perfectly safe and can be repeated many times. Although it is now feasible to detect early inflammatory changes in AS patients using MRI, the cost or even the availability of the procedure may be problematic, limiting its use in everyday practice. In the future, MRI will play an important role in the diagnosis, prognosis, and overall evaluation of the success of treatment for patients with AS.

6

Other Manifestations of Ankylosing Spondylitis

WHILE THE PRIMARY target of AS is the musculoskeletal system, its effects are by no means restricted to the musculoskeletal system. Other organ systems subject to the ravaging effects of AS include the eye (ophthalmologic), the heart (cardiovascular), the lungs (pulmonary), the kidney (renal), the genitourinary tract (reproductive organs and urinary system), the nerves (neurologic) and the gut (gastrointestinal). This chapter explains how AS affects each of these organ systems.

EYE (OPHTHALMOLOGIC)

The most common manifestation of AS in the eye is acute anterior uveitis (AAU), an inflammation of the iris and ciliary body that occurs in the front part of the eye (Figure 6.1). Acute anterior uveitis is also referred to as *iritis*, reflecting the characteristic inflammation of the iris. Anywhere between 25% and 40% of AS patients will develop AAU at some point in their lives. In fact, AAU may even occur before the onset of back pain or even the spine manifestations of AS. In some patients, AAU may be the first sign of the presence of AS. AAU typically affects only one eye at a time, and this fact is important for doctors who see patients with eye inflammation so that the right diagnosis can be made. If the AAU occurs in both eyes at the same time, it may be important to look for another diagnosis.

The likelihood of developing AAU is higher in AS patients with peripheral arthritis. Anterior acute uveitis generally begins with a sudden onset of eye pain, accompanied by redness, extreme sensitivity to light, tearing, and blurred vision. Uveitis lasts several days to weeks, and may reoccur either in the same eye or the opposite eye. Prompt evaluation and institution of treatment by an ophthalmologist is critical to preventing permanent damage to the eye and possible loss of vision. Treatment consists of a steroid medication applied directly to the eye. Emerging research suggests that some of the new biologic agents used to treat AS may aid in the treatment of, and prevent recurrence of, uveitis.

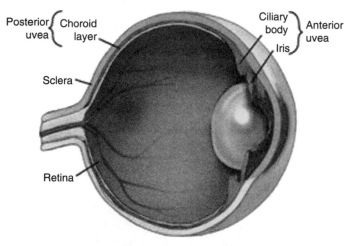

FIGURE 6.1 Anatomy of the Eye

HEART (CARDIOVASCULAR)

Cardiac complications are rare but occur often enough for patients and doctors to be aware of the possibility. They occur after many years of AS, and the majority of patients with AS that experience heart problems are HLA-B27 positive. Types of heart problems include dysfunction of the heart valves, conduction system disturbances, and left ventricular dysfunction. Think of your heart (Figure 6.2) as a complex electrical generator that powers your body. Like the electrical systems in your house or your car, a variety of problems can occur that cause the system to lose power or stop working. Heart valve dysfunction, conduction system disturbances, and left ventricular dysfunction are the equivalent of electrical system power shortages and outages, except that they occur in the heart rather in the car or the house.

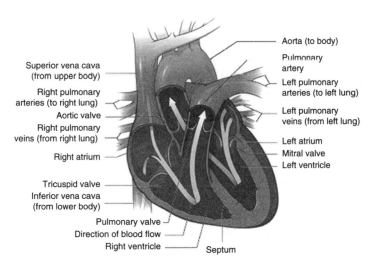

FIGURE 6.2 Anatomy of a Normal Heart

The most common heart valve dysfunction experienced by patients with AS is aortic regurgitation, a condition that occurs in 2%–10% of patients. Aortic regurgitation occurs when the aortic value of the heart weakens and prevents the valve from closing tightly. Blood usually travels from the heart through the aortic valve into the aorta. The aortic valve, while allowing forward flow, usually prevents backflow. As the valve "weakens," some of the forward flowing blood travels back into the heart, which, if severe enough, may lead to heart failure. Severe aortic regurgitation may be treated with valve replacement surgery.

Conduction system disturbances are just that—a disruption of the electrical impulses that power the heart. The frequency of conduction system disturbances in patients with AS ranges from 3% in patients having had the disease for up to 15 years, to 9% in patients having had the disease for up to 30 years. Fortunately, conduction system disturbances are easily managed. If a total disruption of the heart's electrical system occurs, a condition known as complete heart block, recommended treatment is the placement in the heart of a pacemaker. A pacemaker is a small device that provides electrical stimulation and directs the heart's electrical system to function in an almost normal manner.

Left ventricular dysfunction, like valve dysfunction and conduction system disturbances, is a breakdown in the normal functioning of the heart muscle itself—in this case, the left ventricle. A minority of patients with AS will experience left ventricular dysfunction, which, if left untreated, may lead to heart failure, a heart attack, or other types of cardiovascular complications.

LUNGS (PULMONARY)

There is limited information on the prevalence of pulmonary disease in patients with AS. In general, pulmonary complications are not common, but there have been very few studies to give us a true prevalence of this condition in AS. Less severe pulmonary complications include the rigidity of the chest wall that occurs as a result of the forward curvature of the thoracic spine, and inflammation of associated joints that allow the chest wall to expand and fill the lungs with air. The presence of a chest wall with limited expansion and later rigidity is associated with restricted lung function and deep-breathing difficulty. More severe pulmonary complications include obstruction or blockage of the upper airways and acute respiratory failure but these are very rare. Given the fact that AS patients do have restricted chest wall motion that will reduce the ability of lungs to fill with air and clear secretions, it is important for anyone with AS to be vigilant about the possibility of lung infections.

KIDNEY (RENAL)

Kidney problems associated with AS are rare, with the most common complication being secondary amyloidosis. Amyloidosis occurs when too much protein, called *amyloid*, builds up in a particular organ or tissue. Secondary amyloidosis refers to the fact that the build-up of these proteins is related, or secondary, to chronic inflammatory disease, in this case AS. Secondary amyloidosis is more common in Europe than in the United States, and occurs in 1%–3% of patients with AS. Patients with secondary amyloidosis often have proteinuria, an excess of serum proteins that pass from the bloodstream through the kidney into the urine. Urine specimens collected as part of a routine physical examination should be tested for proteinuria. In rare cases, patients may develop kidney problems associated with long-term use of analgesics and nonsteroidal anti-inflammatory drugs.

GENITOURINARY TRACT (REPRODUCTIVE ORGANS AND URINARY SYSTEM)

Ankylosing spondylitis may contribute to sexual dysfunction in men and women. In men, AS may contribute to erectile dysfunction, although the evidence is conflicting and the studies on which the evidence is based had small numbers of AS patients. The causes of erectile dysfunction have been attributed to inflammation, side effects of medications, disturbances of body image, and limited mobility. Limited mobility may also contribute to sexual dysfunction in women, causing painful intercourse. These are issues that are not brought up routinely in doctor visits, but they can be disabling in some circumstances and definitely contribute to a reduced quality of life. Because so much can be done to treat these issues, it is important for AS patients and their spouses to address them during visits to a health care provider.

NERVES (NEUROLOGIC)

Spinal fractures are the most common neurologic complication of AS. That said, spinal fractures occur in only a small percentage of AS patients. The contributing factors and other aspects of spinal fractures are also discussed in Chapter 7. Two of the most frequent types of fractures are vertebral fractures, occurring as a result of ankylosed spines subject to even minor trauma, and stress fractures that occur in the cervicothoracic and thoracolumbar junction. The cervico-thoracic area encompasses the neck and the upper back, and the thoracolumbar junction includes the area where most low back pain is experienced.

Spinal fractures caused by even minor trauma are the most dangerous since they may not be recognized early and sometimes not even noticed by the patient. There may be a sudden loss of height, for example. These fractures can prog-ress quickly if stabilization of the spine does not take place. The spine in AS does not have the ability to withstand forces as a normal spine could do, and even minor trauma can cause this fragile spine to break. In addition, a restricted line of sight caused by a lack of neck mobility could lead to a patient tripping on a step or missing a curb while walking—this could lead to a fall to the ground and a spinal fracture. Most rheumatologists, including the author of this book, highly recommend to their AS patients that they should avoid activ-ities that put them at extreme risk for serious spinal trauma such as snow skiing, skateboarding, or riding a motorcycle.

Irritation of the spinal nerves is another neurological condition that may affect AS patients. This irritation is referred to as *subluxation* and it results when one or more of the bones in the spine move out of position, creating pressure or irritation on the spinal nerves.

A rare but serious complication in patients who have had AS for many years is a slowly progressive *cauda equina* syndrome that can cut off movement and sensation.

Cauda equina syndrome affects the bundle of nerve roots (*cauda equina*) at the lower end of the spinal cord, and occurs when the nerve roots are irritated by inflammation or wrapped by fibrous tissue and compressed. This irritation and compression of the nerve roots may also result in bowel and bladder problems. Symptoms of *cauda equina* include a loss of sensation and motor function in the lower half of the body, and patients experiencing either or both of these should seek immediate treatment.

GUT (GASTROINTESTINAL)

There is a close connection between inflammatory bowel disease (IBD) and AS, although the reasons for this association have not been well established and are currently under investigation. The very latest information about this relationship tells us that there are genes in common between these two conditions. Inflammatory bowel disease is a term used to describe two chronic diseases that cause inflammation of the intestines: ulcerative colitis and Crohn's disease. While most patients with AS do not have either ulcerative colitis or Crohn's disease, about 60% of patients do experience a less severe form of intestinal inflammation, the inflammation of which may resemble Crohn's disease.

The connection between AS and IBD is a complicated one, and is slowly being unraveled in various research laboratories around the world. It is well known, and has been observed for decades, that patients with IBD can evolve into AS, and vice versa. It is also known that patients with AS can have asymptomatic—that is, clinically silent—findings of IBD, if they are carefully examined by upper or lower endoscopy or by sensitive measures that can detect inflammation in the stool of patients with AS. Researchers are now finding antibodies against certain bacteria in AS patients that are usually found in IBD patients. It is hoped that continued research in this area will lead to finding the genetic predisposition and environmental triggers that start and sustain AS.

7

Bone Health

WHEN YOU HEAR the word *osteoporosis* you may think that it is a condition that only occurs in older, postmenopausal women. It is regrettable that television advertising by pharmaceutical companies promotes this sort of public bias and lack of appreciation of the disease as it truly exists in the population. However, osteoporosis—a disease characterized by decreased bone mass and bone density that results in thinning of the bone tissue and weakened bones—occurs in 19%–62% of patients with ankylosing spondylitis, and is associated with an increased risk of vertebral fractures. Over time, men with AS experience an annual total bone mass loss of 2.2%. Spinal osteoporosis is more frequently observed in patients with severe AS, who have had the disease for many years. Surprisingly, osteoporosis occurs in spite of the overgrowth of bone tissue and bone formation that is characteristic of AS. The inflammatory process that occurs as a result of AS is a significant factor contributing to osteoporosis, as are a reduced capacity to absorb shock, and the lack of spinal mobility. Unfortunately, traditional bone density scans used to detect the presence of osteoporosis are not reliable in patients with AS because of the presence of new bone formation associated with the disease, thus making osteoporosis a difficult condition to detect in AS patients.

FRACTURES

An inflexible spine is more likely to fracture when impacted because it is unable to absorb the normal stresses and strains we experience every day. Even a minor slip or fall can cause a fracture in patients with AS—fractures that are not likely to occur in persons with a healthy spine able to absorb the shocks we experience in daily life. For this reason, it is important for patients with AS to avoid activities that might cause severe injury to the spine, such as climbing a ladder or riding a motorcycle. Making adjustments to preserve spine health is a minor inconvenience compared to the magnitude and seriousness of the problem should an injury occur.

Fractures may occur in multiple locations along the vertebral body. Factors associated with the risk of fracture include gender (men are more likely than women to experience fractures); low body weight; low bone mineral density; longer disease duration; extensive syndesmophytes, a bony growth seen in the ligaments of the spine; higher scores on the modified Stoke Ankylosing Spondylitis Spine Score; worse level of disease activity; peripheral joint involvement; restricted spinal movement; and increased occiput-to-wall distance, a measure of thoracic spine extension.

It is often difficult for physicians to diagnosis fractures in patients with AS. There are several reasons for this difficulty. First, the signs and symptoms of vertebral fractures in AS patients differ somewhat from the signs and symptoms typical of fractures in patients without AS. As a result, fractures in AS patients are often attributed to chronic pain and disease activity. Second, fractures often occur in places other than the vertebral body, such as in the vertebral arch and its pedicles, structures that surround the spinal cord and allow the nerves to exit. The location of these fractures makes them difficult to diagnose even with imaging studies. Third, the presence of soft tissue and other bones in the area contribute to less than adequate quality X-ray images, making it difficult to detect the presence of vertebral fractures with the usual conventional radiographs. Finally, researchers have not been able to reach a consensus about the definition of vertebral fractures.

PRESERVING BONE DENSITY

Consuming enough calcium and vitamin D is one way to prevent or delay the possibility of developing osteoporosis and the resulting increased risk of fracture. The recommended daily dose is 1,500 milligrams (mg) for calcium, and 800 IU/day for vitamin D. Dairy products provide the richest source of calcium, although calcium supplements are available over-the-counter. Vitamin D is important because it maximizes the body's absorption of calcium. Our bodies produce vitamin D as a result of exposure to direct sunlight. Sources of vitamin D include milk, cereals fortified with vitamin D, cheese, and egg yolks, as well as over-the-counter supplements and fish oil.

When possible, exercise. Weight-bearing exercise helps to preserve bone mineral density and is essential to maintaining strength and flexibility.

TREATMENT

Fortunately, treatment is available for osteoporosis. Bisphosphonates, a class of drugs that prevent the loss of bone mass, are generally effective in treating osteoporosis. However, there are other choices that are coming on the scene every day. Certain chemicals and biologic drugs will affect different aspects of bone metabolism—some stop the increased or abnormal resorption of bone, while others stimulate bone formation. Some drugs that patients take may affect bone metabolism in ways that may not be readily apparent, but may be detrimental to your health. In addition, there may be side effects caused by treatment of osteoporosis—long-term use of certain of these drugs might actually cause complications that may be difficult to diagnose correctly. Your rheumatologist will develop a treatment protocol that best fits your situation. Bone health is an important part of the management of patients with AS—just as heart health is, or mental health. A rational and scientific assessment of bone health is available for patients with AS—it is a simple matter of asking the right questions and finding the answers.

PART THREE

ASSOCIATED CONDITIONS

THE TWO CHAPTERS in this section—Chapter 8: Juvenile-Onset Ankylosing Spondylitis, and Chapter 9: Spondyloarthritis—are meant primarily for reference. These chapters tell the story of the relationship between ankylosing spondylitis and its manifestation in children, as well as its commonalities with other chronic inflammatory conditions. Feel free to skip these chapters if the information is not directly relevant to your situation.

8

Juvenile-Onset Ankylosing Spondylitis

ANKYLOSING SPONDYLITIS (AS) begins primarily in adolescent and young adult males between the ages of 15 and 25, although it is possible for AS to develop in children and young teens. Ankylosing spondylitis that develops prior to the age of 16 is referred to as juvenile-onset ankylosing spondylitis (JOAS). Symptoms typically occur between the ages of 8 and 12 years. The prevalence of JOAS within the whole spectrum of AS ranges from 9% to 21% in Caucasian populations, and may be as high as 28%–54% in Mexican Mestizo (a mix of Caucasians of Spanish origin and Amerindians).

The cause of JOAS is unknown, although, like AS, the association with the HLA-B27 antigen suggests a strong genetic factor. The HLA-B27 test is positive in over 90% of children with AS. In spite of the fact that there are many similarities between JOAS and AS, some scientists question whether these are the same or fundamentally different conditions. The answer to that question, while beyond the scope of this book, will come in time, as further studies are done on the pathogenesis of the disease.

PRESENTATION AND SYMPTOMS OF JUVENILE-ONSET ANKYLOSING SPONDYLITIS

Enthesitis, pain and tenderness at the entheses, is the most frequent initial manifestation of JOAS. Two-thirds of patients manifest with enthesitis during the first year of the disease, with almost 80% experiencing enthesitis in subsequent years. The primary difference between the clinical presentation of JOAS and that of AS is that JOAS is initially manifest in inflammation in the peripheral joints of the body, especially in the lower extremities, rather than the axial joints of the body, or the spine. Targets of peripheral inflammation include the hip, ankles, knees, and feet. Swelling and redness of the inflamed tissue may, in some cases, be seen in the skin covering the underlying joint disease activity, causing pain and tenderness to touch. Inflammation will continue to cause pain until it is treated. As the disease progresses, the spine will eventually be affected, just as it is in adult AS patients. In the first year after diagnosis, less than 15% of patients with JOAS have axial symptoms. The prevalence of spinal joint pain and stiffness, as well as chest expansion difficulties, increases after 2.5 years of onset and reaches a maximum 5 to 10 years after onset.

The symptoms of JOAS are similar to those of AS and include the following:

- Back pain, usually most severe during sleep or during rest
- Early morning stiffness
- Stooped posture in response to back pain (bending forward tends to relieve the pain)
- Inability to take a deep breath, if the joints between the ribs and spine are affected
- Appetite loss
- Weight loss
- Fatigue
- Fever

- Anemia
- Enthesitis: pain at the site of attachment of muscles, ligaments, and/or tendons to bone
- Joint pain, particularly in the legs
- Vague localized pain, usually in the buttocks, thighs, heels, or near the shoulders
- Eye inflammation that is painful and causes redness and light sensitivity; patients may have frequent recurrences of eye inflammation. This is called uveitis and is discussed in other chapters of this book.

The frequency with which these and other symptoms occur varies. Approximately 5% to 10% of patients with JOAS will have high-grade fever, weight loss, muscle weakness, fatigue, and anemia. About one-fourth of patients will experience an attack of acute uveitis. Although rare, some patients may experience cardiovascular manifestations.

DIAGNOSIS AND TREATMENT OF JUVENILE-ONSET ANKYLOSING SPONDYLITIS

Adult-onset criteria and methodologies are typically used to make a diagnosis of JOAS. As noted in Chapter 5, this includes a complete medical history, physical examination, blood work, and radiographic examination.

The goal of treatment for JOAS is to reduce pain and stiffness, prevent deformities, and ensure that the child with JOAS is able to maintain as normal and active a lifestyle as possible. Although there is no cure for JOAS, it may be possible to slow or prevent disease progression and long-term damage. Specific treatment for JOAS is determined by the physician based on:

- Overall health and medical history
- Extent of the condition
- Tolerance for specific medications, procedures, and therapies
- Expectation for the course of the disease

Treatment may include:

- Nonsteroidal anti-inflammatory drugs (NSAIDs), to reduce pain and inflammation
- Short-term use of corticosteroids (to reduce inflammation)
- Maintenance of proper posture
- Regular exercise, including exercises that strengthen back muscles
- Physical therapy
- New biologic therapies such as anti-TNF agents. These drugs were developed initially for adult AS, and they have shown remarkable benefit in reducing pain and inflammation, increasing mobility, and enhancing quality of life in adults with AS

Caring for a child with JOAS requires a team of dedicated professionals, including a rheumatologist, a physical therapist, a nurse, a psychologist, a nutritionist, and an ophthalmologist. The rheumatologist is there to provide medical treatment, direct the entire team, and assess the child's health status on an ongoing basis. A physical therapist can work with the child and his/her family to develop a safe, effective exercise program that aims to preserve and strengthen physical function. A nurse frequently provides health education to patients and family members, and may serve as a liaison between the physician and patient. The nurse may also be called upon to interface with the child's teachers and school nurses. Children with JOAS face challenges that healthy children do not. As a result, a psychologist may be required to assist the child and/or his/her family to cope with the effects of JOAS. A nutritionist is essential to help the child maintain a healthy weight, as excessive weight gain can stress already inflamed joints. Finally, an ophthalmologist should be consulted at the appearance of any adverse eye symptoms, as patients with JOAS frequently experience uveitis.

9

Spondyloarthritis

ANKYLOSING SPONDYLITIS (AS) is a member of a family of diseases known as *spondyloarthritis* (SpA); these are similar inflammatory rheumatic conditions characterized by involvement of the axial skeleton, peripheral joints, and entheses. These conditions share genetic predisposition, may run together in families and, in fact, sometimes overlap in terms of clinical manifestations and will, in some situations, actually turn into each other over time. Other body parts such as the eyes, skin, gut, and genitourinary tract may also be affected; other chapters of this book will address these conditions. The SpAs are characterized by a strong genetic component (HLA-B27, as well as other newly discovered genes) in addition to painful inflammation. Signs and symptoms of SpA present themselves most often between the ages of 20 and 30 years and, with the exception of psoriatic arthritis, generally occur more frequently in men. In addition to AS, SpAs include: reactive arthritis (ReA); psoriatic arthritis (PsA); enteropathic arthritis; juvenile-onset SpA; and undifferentiated SpA. In the past, spondyloarthritis was sometimes referred to as "seronegative" spondyloarthritis or in some situations they were called "rheumatoid variants," because of the clinical resemblance to rheumatoid arthritis (RA). However, the blood test for rheumatoid factor, an important marker for RA, was always negative in patients with SpA—thus the use of term *seronegative spondyloarthritis*. There are no routine laboratory tests to definitively ascertain the presence of SpA. As a result, a diagnosis of ReA, PsA, enteropathic arthritis, juvenile SpA, or undifferentiated SpA requires the skilled clinical judgment of a rheumatologist due to the several shared characteristics of these conditions as well as their subtle, nuanced differences.

REACTIVE ARTHRITIS

Reactive arthritis (ReA), as the name implies, occurs in reaction to a specific triggering event, in this case a bacterial infection, usually in either the gastrointestinal or urinary tract. There is some speculation that ReA may also occur coincident with the human immunodeficiency virus (HIV) or even other viruses, but there is no definitive proof that there is a viral trigger for most cases. This initial "trigger" of infection may not even be noticed by the patient, or may be dismissed as a minor, inconsequential event. Patients with ReA typically experience pain and swelling in the large joints of the lower body, such as the feet, knees, ankles, and hips. While the pain and inflammation of ReA generally appears in the lower body, it is not uncommon for patients with ReA to experience pain and swelling in the upper body as well. About 30% of patients will have acute low back pain that is worse at night and radiates to the buttocks, similar to the acute low back pain experienced by patients with AS. Other, less common symptoms include conjunctivitis, a swelling or infection of the lining of the eyelid, acute anterior uveitis, and various skin manifestations. These skin manifestations can occur in moist mucous membranes of the mouth, and are usually not symptomatic. Sometimes they may occur in the genitals—on the penis for men or in the vaginal area for women. Because of these lesions on the genitals, these conditions may even be confused with certain other venereal infections which are infections transmitted by sexual activity. Occasionally they may occur on the palms or soles of the feet, and look like eczema or psoriasis.

Reactive arthritis generally occurs in adults between the ages of 30 and 40, usually 1 to 4 weeks following the activating infection. Three of the most common bacteria associated with ReA are *Chlamydia trachomatis,* a type of genital infection transmitted by sexual contact, *Salmonella or Shigella,* a type of severe food poisoning, and *Yersinia,* a gram-negative bacteria also acquired by eating food. Men and women are at equal risk for ReA when the source of infection is gastrointestinal, but men are at greater risk when the source of infection is genitourinary.

The average duration of acute ReA varies from 3 to 5 months. Approximately 4%–19% of patients, depending on the source of the initial infection, will experience an acute episode that lasts longer than one year. There is a genetic component to ReA, with HLA-B27 positive patients being susceptible to having a more severe disease course. Patients with ReA may recover, continue to experience occasional or chronic joint pain, develop chronic arthritis, or progress to AS. Recovery rates and disease progression vary by type of infection. For example, 20% of patients with *Shigella* as the triggering infection recover, versus 45% of patients with *Yersinia.* Up to 68% of patients whose ReA was triggered by *Chlamydia trachomatis* will continue to experience occasional or even chronic joint pain. Severe disability associated with ReA occurs in less than 15% of patients.

Treatment of ReA should target both the initial infection and the attendant arthritis. In many cases, however, it may be difficult to isolate the cause of the initial infection. When it is possible to identify the initial infection, treatment of the infection consists of a course of antibiotics specific to that organism. Initial treatment for the pain and inflammation attendant to ReA is an over-the-counter nonsteroidal anti-inflammatory drug (NSAID) or prescription strength NSAIDs. Pain from arthritis that is not alleviated with an NSAID may be treated with corticosteroid injections if there are only a small number of joints involved. If the condition becomes chronic and the arthritis persists, more aggressive treatments, similar to those employed in AS, are recommended—for example, methotrexate or other disease-modifying antirheumatic drugs (DMARDs). In more severe and chronic cases, biologic drugs may be employed. Patients are advised to minimize use of weight-bearing joints during active ReA.

PSORIATIC ARTHRITIS

Psoriatic arthritis, as its name implies, is an inflammatory arthritis that occurs in individuals with psoriasis. Most of the time psoriasis precedes the arthritis; however, sometimes the arthritis will come first, and psoriasis appears later. Psoriasis is a skin condition in which dead skin cells build up to form thick, dry, scaly patches on the elbows, knees, scalp, or lower spine. Fingernails may become pitted, discolored, and pieces may fall from the nail beds. In general, patients with psoriasis are aware of its presence due to these skin manifestations. However, it is possible for patients to have psoriasis and not be aware of its presence because the psoriasis is hidden in the ear canal, natal cleft, or belly button, for example. It is often difficult to tell the difference between psoriasis and eczema and between poriasis and some other chronic skin conditions such as simple dry skin and dandruff. That is why it is important to see a dermatologist for a diagnosis, and a biopsy of the skin may be necessary to not only make a diagnosis but to rule out other conditions that are confused with psoriasis.

It is estimated that close to 35% of patients with psoriasis will develop PsA, which typically occurs after the onset of psoriasis. That said, 7%–30% of patients may develop PsA prior to the onset of psoriasis, making it more difficult to diagnose. Disease onset is usually between 30 and 50 years of age, with men and women equally affected. Forty percent of patients with PsA report a family history of psoriasis or PsA. This observation has led researchers to search for a genetic predisposition to psoriasis, and some genes have been identified with research ongoing at the present time.

Characteristics of PsA include: joint pain and inflammation; dactylitis (Figure 9.1), a condition in which fingers and toes are very swollen and look like sausages; enthesitis; tensosynovitis, an inflammation of the fluid-filled sheath surrounding a tendon; and sacroiliitis/spondylitis. Fingers and toes are particularly vulnerable. An international group of experts, known as the Classification of Psoriatic Arthritis Study Group, recently developed a set of classification criteria for PsA. A patient with at least three points from the following list is determined to have PsA:

- Current psoriasis or personal or family history of psoriasis (2 points)
- Typical psoriatic nail dystrophy (1 point)
- Dactylitis (1 point)

- Negative test for rheumatoid factor (1 point)
- New bone formation, excluding bone spurs, near or in the region of the joint on radiographs of the hand or foot (1 point)

Unfortunately, PsA is not curable. The goal of treatment is to relieve the pain and swelling that accompany PsA. The first treatment of choice is an NSAID. If an NSAID is not effective in providing significant relief, patients may be prescribed one of several DMARDs such as methotrexate or sulfasalazine. If the condition does not respond to these DMARDs, then a tumor necrosis factor (TNF) inhibitor such as etanercept, infliximab, golimumab, or adalimumab is typically used. It is important to note that these drugs (both DMARDs and anti-TNF agents) will treat both the psoriasis and the arthritis, to a greater or lesser degree for each. In some patients the skin disease will predominate and

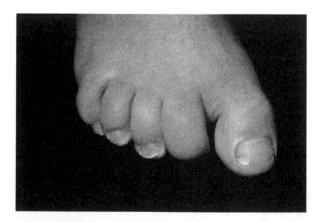

FIGURE 9.1 Dactylitis

determine the need for therapy, but in other patients it is the arthritis that is most disabling and impactful. In addition, there are other biologic drugs that are approved for the psoriasis if the skin disease is particularly severe, but the impact of these drugs on the arthritis is not known and has not been tested. In general, when you are dealing with psoriatic arthritis, there needs to be good communication between rheumatologist and dermatologist in order to produce the most effective therapeutic regimen and meet the needs of the patient. In addition to medical therapy, physical and/or occupational therapy may be prescribed to help protect the affected joints and maintain physical function.

ENTEROPATHIC ARTHRITIS

The term "enteropathy" refers to any disorder of the intestine. Enteropathic arthritis is so named because it is an arthritis associated with Crohn's disease (CD) and ulcerative colitis (UC), both inflammatory bowel diseases (IBD). Up to 20% of patients with CD or UC are afflicted with enteropathic arthritis. In general, but not always, enteropathic arthritis is more active when patients experience an active flare of CD or UC. However, it is possible for enteropathic arthritis to occur prior to, or years following, a diagnosis of inflammatory bowel disease. IBD most commonly begins between the ages of 15 and 35, with men and women being equally susceptible. Symptoms and signs that usually occur with CD include abdominal pain, weight loss, low-grade fever, and diarrhea. Diarrhea and blood loss from the intestine are typical signs and symptoms of UC.

Symptoms of enteropathic arthritis include enthesitis, and pain and swelling in the peripheral joints. Most commonly, the arthritis occurs in the lower limbs. Between 10% and 20% of patients will experience spinal inflammation. Treatment of enteropathic arthritis is slightly different from that of the other SpAs, in that caution is advised relative to the use of NSAIDs because they tend to exacerbate or aggravate gastrointestinal symptoms. The first approach to treating enteropathic arthritis is to treat the IBD, in the hope that treating the IBD will alleviate the patient's arthritis. Peripheral arthritis associated with IBD may be treated with corticosteroids, usually by injection. If relief is not attained through the treatment of the IBD or with corticosteroids for the arthritis, stronger medications, including the use of a tumor necrosis factor (TNF) inhibitor may be advised. Patients with enteropathic arthritis are counseled to seek the care of a rheumatologist and gastroenterologist for optimal disease management. It is not uncommon for patients with enteropathic arthritis to have both conditions (UC or CD alongside either AS or peripheral arthritis) and treatment is guided or dictated by drugs that affect both conditions. Some of the drugs have different therapeutic actions depending on whether the inflammation occurs in the intestine or the joints or both at the same time; the choice of the drug will depend on a lot of factors, some of which have to do with other medications that are needed for the arthritis or the colitis. Therefore, it is necessary to have excellent communication between gastroenterologist and rheumatologist in order to meet the goal of effective and safe management of patients with enteropathic arthritis.

JUVENILE-ONSET SPONDYLOARTHRITIS

This book is focused primarily on the adult manifestations of AS. In order to provide a comprehensive overview of the conditions associated with AS, mention is made here of juvenile-onset spondyloarthritis (SpA). However, the reader is advised to consult other sources for a more in-depth discussion of juvenile-onset SpA.

Juvenile-onset SpA encompasses a range of conditions that begin in children (by definition children have not achieved the age of 18) and have a strong genetic component related to the HLA-B27 allele. While the adult form of SpA usually involves inflammatory low back pain, in children the primary clinical features are enthesitis and arthritis affecting the lower extremities and, in some patients, the sacroiliac and spinal joints. In other words, compared to adults with AS children with this form of SpA will typically present with arthritis of the joints of the lower extremities such as the knees, ankles, or hips. Often an accurate diagnosis is delayed in these children because the spine features of the disease are absent at the beginning. Patients may also experience symptoms involving the skin, eyes, and gut. The prevalence of juvenile-onset SpA is higher in boys than in girls during the prepubescent years, but the proportion of girls with juvenile-onset SpA increases with age and eventually equals the proportion of boys with juvenile-onset SpA. As a consequence of its early age onset, juvenile-onset SpA may result in greater functional and quality-of-life impairment if it becomes a chronic condition. Recent evidence indicates that because of the early involvement of the hip in children with SpA there will be a greater impact on mobility, functional impairment, and quality of life compared to an adult with a similar disease duration.

Given the range of conditions that can occur in children with arthritis, a specific diagnosis of SpA will be dependent upon clinical, laboratory, and radiographic findings, along with the clinical judgment of a pediatric rheumatologist. Consultation and management should involve a multidisciplinary team including rheumatologist, pediatrician, and psychologist. Although there is no cure for juvenile-onset SpA, treatment options are improving in this era of biologic drugs. These agents are employed in the management of childhood onset SpA similar to adult onset AS with very promising results in terms of pain relief and improving functional capacity.

UNDIFFERENTIATED SPONDYLOARTHRITIS

The term *undifferentiated spondyloarthritis* (uSpA) was first used in 1980 to describe a wide variety of spondyloarthritides, with a strong genetic component, that do not meet any of the classification criteria for AS or the SpAs described in this chapter. Undifferentiated SpA is one of the most difficult diseases to diagnose, even for experienced rheumatologists, and patients may experience long delays until a correct diagnosis is made. Some patients diagnosed with uSpA may go on to develop one of the definitive SpAs mentioned in this chapter. Even after diagnosis, patients with uSpA face continued challenges due to the variable nature of the disease course, the severity of the disease itself and, not uncommonly, treatment resistance.

Men are more likely than women to be diagnosed with uSpA. Fifty percent of the time, onset of uSpA occurs during childhood; the average age of onset is between 16 and 23 years of age. The signs and symptoms of uSpA may include any of the signs and symptoms discussed in this chapter, such as dactylitis, enthesitis, and acute anterior uveitis, as well as sacroiliitis and peripheral arthritis. The prevalence of these symptoms varies. For example, at the low end, 4% of patients with uSpA also have IBD. At the high end, 60%–100% of patients have peripheral arthritis.

There is very little data from clinical trials to guide physicians in the treatment of uSpA. For the most part, rheumatologists treat uSpA in the same way they treat AS. Once a diagnosis is made, the treatment decisions are easier and one can expect an excellent outcome from the new biologic agents much as we see in the more differentiated conditions such as psoriatic arthritis, enteropathic arthritis, or even AS.

PART FOUR

DISEASE MANAGEMENT

THE THREE CHAPTERS in this section are designed to help you manage your disease. Chapter 10 addresses medical and non-medical treatment for ankylosing spondylitis (AS), Chapter 11 reviews the types of surgical procedures available to patients with AS, and Chapter 12 provides guidelines for engaging in physical activity and the daily activities of life.

10

Disease Management

UNDERSTANDABLY, YOU ARE concerned about the prospect of living life with ankylosing spondylitis (AS). While it is true that AS is a significant part of your life, it is important to focus on the positive changes you can make that will help you manage and cope with your disease. Rather than letting AS control your life, you need to ask yourself: How can I maximize my physical health and well-being while living with AS? This chapter is intended to provide answers to just such a question.

There are two types of treatments available to you: *non-pharmacologic* treatment, which encompasses patient education, exercise and physical therapy, and *pharmacologic* treatment, the medical term for drug treatment. The objectives of both types of treatment are to minimize pain and stiffness, prevent structural damage and long-term disability, and improve and/or maintain mobility and quality of life. Any treatment plan should be developed in consultation with your rheumatologist and tailored to your individual needs based on your disease activity and severity, symptoms, functional status, structural damage, and current health status. In severe cases, surgery (Chapter 11) may be recommended as an adjunct to treatment.

NONPHARMACOLOGIC TREATMENT

Patient Education

In order for you to take ownership of your disease and learn to control it, rather than letting it control you, you need to be well-informed. Fortunately, there are a wide variety of patient education resources available for AS patients. These resources will provide the information you need to take charge, including learning about implementing a regular exercise program, using complementary treatments such as pain management and relaxation techniques, the appropriate use of aids and devices and, ultimately, the development of an action plan to improve your health and long-term outcomes. In order to take advantage of patient education, you should:

- Request that your rheumatologist and/or physical therapist provide you with pamphlets, books, and video or audiotapes about AS.
- Determine whether there are any AS support groups in your area.
- Take advantage of the Internet to visit web sites such as the Spondylitis Association of America (www.spondylitis.org) or the Ankylosing Spondylitis International Federation (www.asif.rheumanet.org and www.spondylitis-international.org) that provide extensive resources to help patients manage their disease.

Exercise and Physical Therapy

The adoption and maintenance of a regular exercise routine is crucial for patients with AS, the benefits of which include less pain, improved posture, enhanced chest expansion, and increased lung capacity. Your personal preference will determine whether to exercise alone, with a group, or with a physical therapist. Regardless of your preference, though, it is imperative that you consult with both your rheumatologist

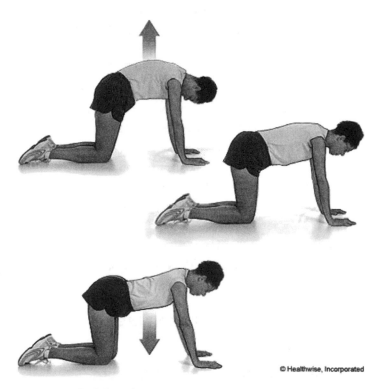

FIGURE 10.1 Back Stretches

1. Get down on your hands and knees on the floor.
2. Relax your head and allow it to droop.
3. Round your back up toward the ceiling until you feel a nice stretch in your upper, middle, and lower back.
4. Hold this stretch for as long as it feels comfortable, or about 15 to 30 seconds.
5. Return to the starting position with a flat back while you are on all fours.
6. Let your back sway by pressing your stomach toward the floor. Lift your buttocks toward the ceiling.
7. Hold each position for 15 to 30 seconds.
8. Repeat 2 to 4 times.

and physical therapist about the best exercise program for you. Should you choose to exercise on your own, swimming, water aerobics, or a stationary bicycle are excellent choices. Activities to be avoided include high-impact and contact sports, as well as any exercise that involves abrupt movement of the spine. Physical therapy is an excellent way to establish a long-term exercise routine, and a physical therapist can provide you with specific recommendations such as exercises for spinal extension, deep breathing, and improved range of motion for your back (Figure 10.1), neck, shoulders, and hips.

PHARMACOLOGIC TREATMENT

Nonsteroidal Anti-Inflammatory Drugs

The first choice drug therapy for patients with AS is a nonsteroidal anti-inflammatory drug (NSAID). There are more than 20 types of NSAIDs currently available; two that may be most familiar are ibuprofen (Advil, Motrin) and naproxen (Aleve, Naprosyn). A NSAID will reduce the pain and inflammation associated with AS but it does not cure the disease. Some NSAIDs are designed to be taken several times a day, while other, longer-acting types are designed to be taken only once or twice a day. The choice of drug as well as its dose and frequency of administration should be determined by discussions with your rheumatologist. In general, individuals will vary in their responses to different drugs, and there is no "one size fits all" approach with these agents. In other words, there is no one of these drugs that has been shown to be any better than any other and it entirely depends on the individual's own response to each drug, which will vary from patient to patient. The choice also depends on what other drugs the patient is taking and whether or not there are risk factors for toxicity for individual agents.

Although NSAIDs are safe and effective, they are not without side effects. Ten percent to 60% of patients taking NSAIDs experience minor gastrointestinal symptoms such as nausea, diarrhea, or gastric pain. These symptoms are usually reversible after discontinuing the drug. If they do not go away quickly, then your doctor needs to be consulted for further discussions about why this is happening. Another 1%–2% of patients experience severe side effects after 3 months of use, including ulcers and gastrointestinal bleeding. These signs of toxicity are clearly more serious and immediate medical attention is required. In general, most people will be able to tolerate these drugs without a problem and the rheumatologist relies on symptom evaluation to monitor side effects. However, there are some patients who are at a higher risk for the more serious side effects, and these risks include, but are not limited to, a past history of intolerance to previous use of these drugs, concomitant use of corticosteroids, older age of the patient, use of anticoagulants, and the presence of other underlying diseases such as diabetes mellitus, heart disease, and hypertension. It is important that long-term use of NSAIDs be carefully monitored by your rheumatologist. There may be a variety of ways that these drugs will still be employed but the safety risk can be reduced.

Corticosteroids

Corticosteroids are powerful anti-inflammatory agents and when used long term, in any form, they can suppress the immune system and cause unwanted side effects. Some of these side effects are permanent and not readily reversible. As a result of this caution, they are not routinely used in the treatment of AS. An expert review panel notes that "corticosteroid injections directed to the local site of musculoskeletal inflammation may be considered, but the use of systemic corticosteroids for axial disease is not supported by the available evidence."[1] There may be occasions, however, when your physician determines that corticosteroids are beneficial, such as during a particularly active time or major flare. Corticosteroids may be administered intravenously, that is, directly into the vein, or by injection intra-muscularly, deep below the skin. Mostly, however, they are taken by mouth if used for systemic

---

1. Zochling J, van der Heijde D, Burgos-Vargas R, et al. ASAS/EULAR recommendations for the management of ankylosing spondylitis. *Ann Rheum Dis* 2006;65:442–452.

inflammation. On occasion, corticosteroids can be injected directly into the sacroiliac joints under imaging guidance by an experienced practitioner. The problem with this approach is that the benefit is most likely short-lived, and repeated corticosteroid injections into inflamed joints is not recommended for regular long term care of the disease.

Bisphosphonates

Bisphosphonates are a class of drugs that are used to prevent the loss of bone mass. They are not specifically used to treat AS, but merit a brief mention here because they are used to treat osteoporosis, a not uncommon side effect of AS. Osteoporosis can be a concomitant and severe complication of AS and can even increase the risk of a spinal fracture in this disease. Therefore it is important that the bone health of any patient with AS be evaluated not only at the outset of disease but along the way as well. Bisphosphonates may be utilized in AS patients to treat osteoporosis and assist in fracture prevention, but their administration needs careful consideration of risk and benefit in the individual patient. A discussion of this issue should take place with your physician on a regular basis.

Disease-modifying Antirheumatic Drugs

Treatment with medication stronger than a NSAID may be necessary in up to half of all patients with AS. Although routinely used in the treatment of rheumatoid arthritis (RA), disease-modifying antirheumatic drugs (DMARDs) are less frequently used to treat AS patients. The two most frequently used DMARDs for RA are methotrexate and sulfasalazine, both slow-acting compounds that may require use over several months before any relief is felt. There is little evidence to support the use of either of these drugs to treat the spinal disease in AS patients. However, there is some evidence that both of these agents can be employed to treat the peripheral arthritis that occurs in patients with AS, psoriatic arthritis, enteropathic arthritis, or undifferentiated SpA. Serious side effects are rarely encountered with the use of these drugs, but occasional allergic reactions are encountered and regular monitoring is required.

Tumor Necrosis Factor-alpha Inhibitors

The introduction of tumor necrosis factor-alpha (TNF-α) inhibitor therapy for the treatment of AS is one of the most remarkable achievements to date in the management of this complex condition. TNF-α inhibitors are a class of therapeutics known as *biologics* that work to block the inflammatory response evoked by a type of cytokine known as tumor necrosis factor. Normally, TNF serves a protective function by massing inflammatory cells to fight infection. In patients with AS, though, TNF is present in excess, causing pain and inflammation.

There are currently four types of TNF-α inhibitors approved by the U.S. Food and Drug Administration for use in patients with AS or psoriatic arthritis. They are: etanercept (Enbrel), infliximab (Remicade), golimumab (Simponi), and adalimumab (Humira). In clinical trials, patients receiving treatment with a TNF-α inhibitor showed significant improvement in back pain, stiffness, peripheral arthritis, and enthesitis when compared to a control (untreated) group.

Treatment with a TNF-α inhibitor is a long-term proposition and is not without risks. Side effects that are reported include allergic reactions at the infusion or injection site, an increased risk of infection, congestive heart failure, lymphoma, skin cancers, or solid organ cancers. Much of the information we have about the risks and side effects of these drugs comes from studies of the effectiveness of TNF-α inhibitors in rheumatoid arthritis (RA). It is a fact that patients with RA have an increased incidence of these adverse events even without taking these drugs. With AS, we do not know for sure whether there is an increased incidence of these adverse events (infections, malignancies) in the absence of TNF-α inhibitors. Therefore, the question about an increased risk of adverse events in AS patients taking TNF-α inhibitors is not completely answered. Nevertheless, we are being cautious in the warnings about these issues in AS patients because we simply do not know, as yet, if these drugs are safe from these unwanted risks or whether the risk is the same as in RA.

11

Surgery

THE GOOD NEWS is that most patients with ankylosing spondylitis (AS) do not require surgery during the course of their lifetime. The bad news is that spine surgery or joint replacement surgery may be necessary in cases of severe disease activity that goes on unchecked and produces damage that is not reversible. In addition, there is always the possibility that trauma can cause problems that can only be addressed by surgery. Spine surgery may be required when the patient has severe spinal deformity, traumatic or spinal instability, or neurologic deficits, such as weakness or numbness. Joint replacement surgery may be necessary when hip or knee joints have become so damaged by disease that they need to be replaced. While all surgery entails some amount of risk, patients with AS undergoing any type of surgical procedure pose unique challenges for the surgeon and anesthesiologist.

SPINE SURGERY

There are several types of spine surgeries used to treat AS. When surgery is indicated, the type of surgery performed will depend on several factors including patient's age, and location and severity of the deformity or damage. Spine surgeries for AS patients include osteotomy, decompression, and spinal instrumentation and fusion. An osteotomy is used to correct spinal deformities by cutting and realigning the bone. In some cases, spinal instrumentation and fusion may be performed at the same time as the osteotomy in order to stabilize the spine during the healing process. Decompression surgery is a general term that refers to any surgery that involves taking the pressure off the spinal cord or nerves to restore neurologic function or prevent neurologic dysfunction. Spinal instrumentation and fusion are designed to correct spinal deformities and stabilize the spinal column. Instrumentation involves the use of medical hardware such as rods, bars, wires, and screws, whereas fusion uses bone graft to stimulate two bony surfaces to grow together. Following surgery in the spine, a halo brace may be required to immobilize the spine during the healing process. Patients requiring spine surgery should receive a thorough consultation and evaluation with an experienced spine surgeon (usually either an orthopedist or a neurosurgeon), who will recommend the most appropriate surgery.

JOINT REPLACEMENT

Hips and knees are the most common joints requiring replacement in patients with AS. Joint replacement surgery may be indicated when the patient's functioning has been severely impacted or pain in the affected joint becomes intolerable. It is recommended that the determination of whether joint replacement surgery should be performed be a mutual decision between patient, rheumatologist, and orthopedic surgeon. In addition to pain and functional limitations, the decision to perform joint replacement surgery should include a discussion of the cost of the procedure, risk factors, and recovery time, including any necessary physical therapy.

Both hip and knee replacement surgery require the removal of the existing skeletal structure and replacement with an artificial structure. In the case of a hip replacement, the bone and cartilage on the ball-and-socket hip joint is removed and replaced with an artificial hip (Figure 11.1) that serves the same function. During a knee replacement, the bone and cartilage on the end of the thigh bone and the top of the shin bone are removed and replaced with a metal or plastic knee (Figure 11.2).

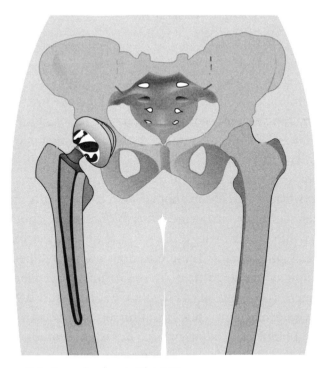

FIGURE 11.1 Example of an Artificial Hip

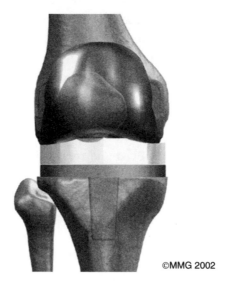

©MMG 2002

FIGURE 11.2   Knee Arthroplasty

While joint replacement surgery is quite safe in modern times, artificial joints are still susceptible to infection both immediately following, and for several years after, surgery. Infections are rare, developing in 0.5%–1% of patients in the general population with replacement joints. Infections may occur when bacteria from another source, such as the mouth or genitourinary area, enters the bloodstream and then lodges into an area where there is a foreign object like an artificial joint surface. These infections are very difficult to diagnose as well as to treat. The most important aspect of treatment is prevention. As a result, patients with AS who have undergone joint replacement surgery may be advised to take antibiotic medication prior to dental procedures, gynecologic examination, or prior to any surgery.

SURGICAL CHALLENGES

Patients with AS who undergo spine, joint replacement, or any other type of surgery, pose special challenges for the surgeon and anesthesiologist due to restricted chest capacity, a rigid spine, and compromised jaw-opening capacity. Restricted chest capacity may lead to pulmonary (lung) complications during surgery, and postsurgical lung complications. A rigid spine and compromised jaw-opening capacity make it very difficult for an anesthesiologist to insert a breathing tube into the trachea to keep the airways open during general anesthesia. Consultation with an anesthesiologist prior to surgery is critical, because not all healthcare providers are aware of the surgical limitations involved in treating patients with AS. These challenges may sound frightening; be reassured that while challenging, they are not insurmountable.

12

Physical and Daily Activity

THE PREVIOUS TWO CHAPTERS reviewed various treatment strategies for ankylosing spondylitis (AS): Chapter 10 examined in detail pharmacologic and nonpharmacologic treatments, and Chapter 11 discussed surgical treatment. In this chapter, information is provided on types of physical activity that you can engage in to manage the effects of AS. In addition, recommendations are provided that will help you to accommodate activities of daily life that most people without AS take for granted. While specific treatment recommendations should be provided by your rheumatologist and other members of your healthcare team, in general, as part of your routine it is important to:

- Follow a safe program of daily activity that builds strength and encourages flexibility.
- Adjust your daily activity as needed to avoid excessive pain—know your limitations.
- Eat a healthy diet that includes plenty of fruits and vegetables. Avoid unnecessary carbohydrates. A carbohydrate-rich diet may contribute to being overweight; excess pounds place an unnecessary burden on your spine and other joints.
- Follow your medication schedule.
- Consult frequently with your doctor about questions you have concerning your condition, medication, or any physical concerns.

- Listen to your body and learn to recognize signs of stress and fatigue that may exacerbate AS flares.
- Communicate with family and friends about your AS so that they understand your condition and learn to support your efforts to maintain an active lifestyle and daily activities.

PHYSICAL ACTIVITY

It is of the utmost importance that you begin and maintain a regular exercise program as part of managing your AS. The goal of regular exercise is to prevent further damage from accruing and, for many people, there is an added psychological benefit that comes with regular exercise. Flexing, stretching, deep breathing, side bends, waist turns, and neck stretches and tilts should be included in your core exercise program. Examples of controlled stretching and deep breathing exercises are provided below. Other beneficial exercises include yoga, water therapy, swimming, tai chi, biking, and weight training. The web site of the Spondylitis Association of America (www.spondylitis.org) includes several articles that outline exercises for patients with AS. As mentioned in Chapter 10, it is important for you to consult with a physical therapist and your rheumatologist prior to beginning any exercise program, as they are the persons most familiar with your disease and your specific abilities and limitations.

Controlled stretch (standing). Stand with your heels and buttocks against a wall. Try to flatten your shoulder blades to the wall and gently press the back of your head to touch the wall, keeping your chin down. Hold for a count of five and then relax. Repeat 10 times. Add to this exercise by raising your right arm forward and upward with the elbow straight, your upper arm close to your ear and your thumb toward the wall. Hold for a count of five and then lower. Repeat with the left arm. Repeat 5 times with each arm.

Deep breathing. Rest your hands on the lower part of your rib cage, just above your waist. Breathe in slowly through your nose, filling your lungs with air. Feel your rib cage expand up and outwards. You may also feel your abdomen (stomach muscles) expand as you breathe in. Breathe out slowly through your mouth. Feel your ribs move down and inwards. You can draw in your abdominals as you breathe out. Repeat 5–10 times. Don't hold your breath. Stop if you start to feel dizzy. *You can also practice this exercise lying flat on your back with your knees bent and feet flat on the floor or bed.*

One of the keys to maintaining a regular exercise program is to make sure that you exercise at a time of day that is most convenient for you. If you are stiff when you wake up in the morning, you may want to begin the day with some stretching exercises to loosen your muscles, and wait until later in the day or evening, when you are more comfortable, to complete your remaining exercises. If you are exercising at home, be sure to exercise where it is comfortable–either on a carpeted floor or an exercise mat.

At this point, a note of caution is in order. While you should make every effort to participate in physical activity, it is important for you to realize that because of your AS, you do not have normal spine biomechanics. Your spine is rigid and has lost its ability to function as a "shock absorber," thus making you more prone to injury, such as spinal fractures. Therefore, you must be extremely cautious about performing risky physical activity. Those risky physical activities may be indirect—by exposing yourself to injury from the actions of others. For example, you might be an expert in snow skiing, and perform your activities very carefully. However, the people around you on the slopes will not be as careful and they could run into you, knock you down, or even worse things can be imagined. So, be careful of your environment and the behavior of others, and reduce the risk of injury as much as you can.

THE WORKPLACE

If you are currently employed, you may be concerned about your ability to continue working. Rest assured that the majority of people with AS are able to continue working. In the United States, about 10% of patients with AS discontinue work at 10 years following diagnosis, and another 10% discontinue work at 20 years following diagnosis. The severity of your disease and the type of work in which you are engaged are factors that will determine the type of accommodations, if any, you may need to make in order to continue working.

If you have a desk job, you will want to make sure that you take breaks throughout the day to stretch. While sitting at your desk, make sure that you always sit up straight, and that you do not spend long periods of time with your head bent forward. When using a computer you should be aware of the possibility of unnecessarily bending forward; desks and computer equipment can be arranged in an ergonomically advantageous position. If your job requires you to stand for long periods of time or engage in heavy lifting, you may want to consult with a physical therapist to discuss how you can safely manage your work activities. In addition, you may want to speak directly with your employer about whether any adjustments can be made to accommodate your workload to your limitations. Finally, while this may be more difficult to do, you may want to consider another type of work if too much strain is placed on your spine and hips.

FATIGUE

Fatigue is a major issue for up to 65% of patients with AS at various times during the course of their disease. Women report fatigue more often than men, as do patients with more severe disease. Fatigue contributes to time away from work, decreases ability to function on a daily basis, and limits one's ability to exercise. Causes of fatigue include loss of sleep due to physical discomfort and the inflammation associated with AS. It may be difficult to believe, but our bodies actually use energy while fighting inflammation. At the same time, some of the substances produced during the immune system's response to the inflammatory process are thought to contribute to fatigue. It is important to speak with your rheumatologist if you are experiencing debilitating episodes of fatigue.

RECREATIONAL ACTIVITIES

Recreational activities are just as important for patients with AS as they are for people without AS because they provide a time to get together with family and friends. Recreation is essential to good health, and should be continued as long as you are able to meet the physical demands of any recreational activity in which you are engaged. You may want to check with your rheumatologist, physical therapist, or local AS organization to determine whether there are any sports teams in your area for people with AS.

CHILDREN

Children who are old enough to understand should be provided with factual information about AS. While we often underestimate our children's ability to understand, they may be acutely aware of what is going on with their parents and know more than we think they do. Giving them information about your condition may help to alleviate any anxiety they may feel about having a parent with AS.

If you are caring for an infant, toddler, or young child, you may find that you need to take certain precautions. For example, the handles on a stroller can be adjusted so that you do not stoop while pushing the stroller. Similarly, you may find it easier to bathe an infant in the sink rather than the bathtub so that you are not straining your back leaning over the bathtub.

AUTOMOBILE SAFETY

You do not need to give up driving as a result of having AS. However, you should be aware of steps you can take to make driving easier for you. First, always wear your seatbelt and use proper head, neck, and back support. Second, you may want to install wide-angled side view mirrors on your car, as these mirrors will increase your peripheral vision and make driving easier. Third, if you find it necessary to drive for long periods of time, you may want to stop every hour or two to take a short walk and stretch your back. Finally, if neck stiffness and rigidity make it difficult for you to back your car out of your garage or public parking spaces, you can have special mirrors installed to make these tasks easier for you. Handicap parking places are designed for people with a variety of physical limitations to their driving and parking. These parking spaces are generally in proximity to the places where you want to go. It is important to take advantage of these spaces since they will make parking easier and safer for you and your automobile. It is always a difficult decision to make use of this opportunity because of the stigma associated with being "handicapped," but there is a reason for the laws that permit their existence. Since parking a car today is more frightening than ever before with tight parking spaces and aggressive motorists on the road, it makes sense to be smart and use what is designed only to help.

SMOKING

If you currently smoke cigarettes, it is highly recommended that you quit. Smoking contributes to a wide variety of diseases, and patients with AS are at an increased risk for respiratory complications due to an already compromised pulmonary system. Current research supports the view that cigarette smoking contributes not only to the susceptibility to a variety of arthritis conditions, but it contributes to their severity as well. We don't really know the reasons why this happens, but there is no doubt that it does.

POSTURE

It is critically important for you to maintain good posture at all times, and to stand as tall and as erect as possible. During the day, you should walk and stand as if your back is up against the wall at all times. At night, you should sleep on a firm mattress; sleep on your stomach as much as possible as this position emphasizes extension of the spine. Try sleeping without a pillow.

PART FIVE

THE FUTURE

THESE LAST TWO CHAPTERS summarize the current state of our knowledge about the causes and treatment of AS, identify areas for future research, and provide answers to questions frequently asked by patients with AS.

13

What Does the Future Hold?

LOOKING BACK at the previous chapters in this book tells us that there is much that we do know about ankylosing spondylitis (AS). Specifically, AS is an inflammatory arthritis belonging to a family of conditions known as spondyloarthritis (SpA). Ankylosing spondylitis is characterized by axial skeletal inflammation, enthesitis, and a genetic component dominated by the HLA-B27 gene; it is more prevalent in men, and disease onset occurs during youth and into the prime of life. Primary treatment for AS consists of nonsteroidal anti-inflammatory drugs (NSAIDs) to reduce inflammation, and tumor necrosis factor-alpha (TNF-α) inhibitors to reduce inflammation even more and to improve functional ability. In rare cases, spinal surgery or joint replacement surgery may be necessary to heal fractures, to correct severe deformities, or replace damaged joints. While there is much that we do know about AS, many questions remain unanswered.

First, HLA-B27 appears to be a necessary, but not sufficient, condition for developing AS. Does this signify that other genes are instrumental in the onset of AS?

Second, little is known about the factors that influence the severity and progression of spinal arthritis in patients with AS. Why does one patient progress to fusion of the spine with severe limitations of motion while another patient, even in the same family, progresses slowly if at all and not have any limitations? At the present time, there are no known factors that influence the severity of spinal inflammation or the rate of progression of spinal ankylosis, although we do know that functional disability occurs more quickly in older patients and smokers, and less quickly in patients who do back exercises on a regular basis and have better social support structures. We suspect that genetics have a great deal to do with this variability in progression and outcome, but the studies to examine this hypothesis are just beginning. How can we identify factors that influence the severity of spinal inflammation and functional disability, and potentially leverage that knowledge to develop pharmacologic and genetic treatments to slow the progression and severity of AS?

Third, what is the relationship between inflammation and disease activity? If we can calm the inflammation, can we tame the disease activity? How does pharmacologic treatment affect inflammation and physical function?

Fourth, can new bone formation be stopped or retarded?

Finally, will learning more about the relationship between inflammatory bowel disease (IBD) and AS enable researchers to identify patients at risk for AS prior to disease onset? Or, can an understanding of the relationship between IBD and AS facilitate an earlier diagnosis of AS? The answers to many of these questions hinge on the science of genetics.

The science of genetics is the science of heredity—that is, the traits and characteristics that we inherit from our parents. Genes are the mechanism by which hereditary material is transmitted from generation to generation. The first gene identified to be strongly associated with the development of AS was HLA-B27, and this information was first published in the early 70s. Although, on average, 7% of the general population has the HLA-B27 gene, with the percentage varying among ethnic groups, more than 90% of AS patients are positive for the HLA-B27 gene. Scientists estimate that

20%–50% of genetic susceptibility is accounted for by the HLA-B27 gene. This suggests an answer to the first question we posed—are other genes involved in the onset of AS? Due to the fact that less than half of genetic susceptibility is accounted for by the HLA-B27 gene, there must be other genes involved in the development of AS. Within the last several years, several new genes have been identified as being associated with AS: these include ERAP1, also known as endoplasmic reticulum aminopeptidase 1, and the IL-23R gene, also known as interleukin-23 receptor. More recently, in addition to these, the anthraxin receptor 2 (ANTXR2) and the interleukin 1 receptor 2 (IL1R2) have been implicated in AS susceptibility, as well as "gene deserts" on chromosome 2 at position p15, and on chromosome 21 at the q22 position. These new genes, along with HLA-B27, account for 50% of the genetic risk for AS. In the future, it may be possible to use genetic testing to identify AS susceptibility—in turn, enabling physicians to make an earlier diagnosis of AS, and thereby helping future AS patients to avoid incurring continued damage while waiting for a diagnosis to be made. In spite of the fact that significant scientific discoveries have been made relative to the identification of AS susceptibility genes, there is still much work to be done to learn how, and if, these genes interact with each other, how genes interact with environmental factors to activate AS, and the biologic mechanisms by which these genes facilitate the onset of AS.

While genes strongly determine whether one is likely to get AS, there is very little information available at the present time with which to answer our second set of questions: What factors influence the severity of spinal inflammation, and how can we leverage knowledge of these factors to develop pharmacologic treatments to slow the progression and severity of AS? Research is currently underway at institutions across the country, and throughout the world, to identify factors associated with spinal inflammation, disease progression, and functional limitation. One theory being explored is that it is the inflammation itself that initiates and then sets in motion the process of ankylosis, as a result of a molecularly based trigger. According to this theory, AS is not a disease manifesting with ankylosis as a primary event, but rather a condition where a chronic inflammatory process in the spine results in ankylosis through very complicated, and as yet undiscovered, mechanisms. If researchers are able to identify the biologic mechanisms that trigger and perpetuate the inflammation we see in AS patients, then new treatments can be developed to arrest those mechanisms and slow or delay the inflammatory process. However, there are other theories about how and why bone ankylosis occurs in AS. Based on emerging clinical research observations and basic science studies using animal models, bone growth in AS may result from mechanisms that are unrelated to inflammatory processes. Patients with AS may have aggressive bone production through pathways that are determined by these independent forces, perhaps under genetic control. These areas of research are being explored at the present time.

Our third set of questions about the relationship between inflammation and disease activity is similar, but slightly different than our second set of questions. Here, we are not asking how and why the disease progresses, but rather whether currently available drug treatment is effective at reducing inflammation and disease activity. The good news is that NSAIDs are quite effective in reducing inflammation; the better news is that anti-TNF therapy improves physical function, back pain, flares of uveitis, disturbed sleep, and overall quality of life. It is a stronger weapon against inflammation compared to NSAIDs.

In our fourth question, we ask whether new bone formation that results in ankylosis can be stopped or retarded. The answer is that based on the currently available evidence, we cannot stop or retard new bone formation, even with the recent addition of anti-TNF therapy for the treatment of AS. Studies have shown that over a 2-year period, anti-TNF therapy did not stop the radiographic progression of AS. What does it mean, then, that inflammation and physical function are improved with the use of anti-TNF therapy, but the formation of new bone growth cannot be stopped? What this tells us is two things. The first is that bony overgrowth itself may not be the primary driver of poor physical function or quality of life. The second is that bony overgrowth, and in some cases ankylosis, may be part of the healing process during the time inflammation is controlled by certain agents. This is consistent with the theory mentioned earlier that postulates that AS is a condition where a chronic inflammatory process in the spine results in ankylosis in spite of the fact that inflammation is controlled, and healing takes place through as yet undiscovered mechanisms. Additional research efforts such as imaging studies, laboratory investigations that include studies using animal models of disease, and clinical trials are required before we can definitely determine the relationship between inflammation, new bone growth, and control of symptoms, as well as disease progression and disease activity.

Our final set of questions is related to the apparent link between IBD and AS. Keep in mind that about 10% of patients with AS also have IBD, and that 70% of patients with AS have a subclinical, or mild, case of IBD. Furthermore, scientists have recently discovered that there is a strong genetic link between AS and IBD; this link suggests a common etiology for both diseases. Scientists are continuing to explore the commonalities between AS and IBD in the hope of developing earlier detection methods for the diagnosis of AS. In addition, the study of IBD in association with AS will potentially provide us with insights into finding a potential trigger for AS that resides in the gut. Since scientists know that immune dysregulation occurring in the gut may actually facilitate patients getting IBD, perhaps triggered by micro-organisms that live in the intestines, ongoing research is in progress to determine whether these same mechanisms may be operative in AS. Finding the elusive trigger for AS that starts the disease in the genetically susceptible host is the holy grail of research in AS.

In conclusion, over the past several decades, researchers have identified effective treatments to alleviate the signs and symptoms of AS. In spite of our current fund of knowledge, challenges remain. Overcoming these challenges and identifying disease pathways and genetic mechanisms offer our best hope for developing new and better targeted treatments to enable AS patients to live fully functional lives. Ultimately, the knowledge that is gained by these efforts will give us prevention strategies to either not encounter the disease at all at best, or, at the very least stop it from progressing once it starts.

14

Frequently Asked Questions

A SUBSTANTIAL AMOUNT of material has been covered in this book, ranging from the epidemiology of ankylosing spondylitis (AS) to the structure of the spinal column and bone health; from the characteristics of AS to disease management. Even with all of the information in this book, you may be left with unanswered questions. Ankylosing spondylitis is a serious but manageable condition. Therefore, it is important that you discuss any questions, concerns, or issues that you have with your rheumatologist as he/she is the person most familiar with the details of your particular case. While other sources of information are available—for example, from patient education pamphlets, patient support groups such as the Spondylitis Association of America (SAA), and web sites devoted to AS—only your physician can determine how any particular treatment strategy will apply to you personally. That said, here are some of the most frequently asked questions by patients with AS.

> **Question:** What is the best way for me to communicate with my doctor about questions I have concerning AS?
>
> **Answer:** It is generally best to ask your doctor to answer your questions during the course of your regularly scheduled office visit. You should keep a written list of questions that occur to you prior to your scheduled visit, and bring that list with you to your visit. Those questions will serve as a reminder to you to try to

obtain the information you are concerned about. During your doctor's visit, it is certainly reasonable to make notes about the answers from your doctor regarding each question so that you don't forget important information. If you have any questions about the medical terminology used by your doctor, make sure you ask him/her to explain any words that you do not understand. However, not every question can be answered each time you visit the doctor—there may be issues involving your disease that may take priority during any given visit. Since the disease and your needs will change over time, it is best to establish a good working relationship with your doctor so that you and your doctor are comfortable asking and answering questions on an ongoing basis. Just running through a list of questions in an anxious manner might not be the optimal way to spend time during an office visit—both the doctor and the patient should prioritize the issues that are pertinent to any given visit. Sometimes bringing a family member to the visit as a reminder or a scribe will help—you cannot be expected to remember exactly all of what went on at the visit so it is very useful to have someone to corroborate the story and serve as a source of back up information.

On occasion, it may be necessary or important for you to call your doctor immediately and not wait for a scheduled visit to receive an answer to a question. For example, if you have a sudden increase in pain, or believe that you may have injured yourself, you need to call your doctor immediately.

Question: Do I need to tell my doctor about other prescription medications or dietary supplements that I am taking?

Answer: Yes. Prescription medications, nonprescription medications and dietary supplements, including vitamins and herbal products, are not without risk. When multiple medications are involved, there is always the possibility for an adverse effect due to a drug–drug interaction. As a result, it is important that each of your doctors is familiar with all of your medications. You should review your medication schedule with your doctor at every appointment. This is best done by providing your doctor with a written list of all of your medications. Even though your doctor keeps a record of what was prescribed at your last visit, things change between visits; providing an updated list of your medications at each visit is very important. Maybe you have seen another doctor in the meantime for what seems like an unrelated problem and a drug regimen is changed or altered. For these reasons, you should always hand a list of your current medications to the doctor or his/her staff.

Question: I know that my cigarette smoking is not good for me, but are the consequences worse for someone with AS?

Answer: Yes. There are multiple reasons that the consequences of smoking are worse for patients with AS. First, the evidence is quite clear that patients with AS who smoke experience an increase in disease activity and a decrease in functional ability compared to patients with AS who don't smoke. Second, in addition to the fact that cigarette smoking causes lung irritation and loss of elasticity of the lung tissue, smoking makes breathing even more difficult in AS patients with restricted chest movement. Third, recent studies suggest that patients with AS who smoke do not respond as well to the antitumor necrosis factor (TNF) therapy, one of the primary treatments used to control disease activity. Finally, one of the major risk factors for osteoporosis, a thinning of the bones, is smoking. Patients with AS are already at increased risk for osteoporosis, and smoking only exacerbates that risk.

Question: My doctor has mentioned the possibility that as a consequence of having AS, my eyes may become inflamed. Can you tell me something about this eye inflammation?

Answer: The term for the eye inflammation to which your doctor is referring is *uveitis*. During an attack of uveitis, the uvea, the middle layer of the eye, becomes swollen and irritated. Symptoms of uveitis include blurred vision, eye pain, dark floating spots in your line of sight, redness of the eye, and extreme sensitivity to light. Uveitis is generally treated with steroid eye drops. If you suspect that you are experiencing the onset of uveitis, you should immediately contact your ophthalmologist. If you do not have an ophthalmologist, call your rheumatologist and ask for a recommendation. Do not delay seeking treatment. If diagnosed and treated early, you should not experience any permanent eye damage. If left untreated, you may have permanent eye damage. It is possible for uveitis to reoccur.

Question: Is it safe for a woman with AS to become pregnant—safe for the growing fetus as well as the mother-to-be?

Question: Will my baby inherit AS?

Answer: It is definitely safe for a woman with AS to become pregnant. It is also safe for the fetus, although there is the possibility that the child may develop AS later in his/her life due to the hereditary nature of the disease. While there is a 50% chance of the newborn inheriting the HLA-B27 gene, the chance of actually developing AS ranges from 5% to 20% if the gene is inherited.

During pregnancy, about 50% of pregnant women with AS show no change in AS symptoms, about 25% show a decrease in AS symptoms, and the remaining 25% show an increase in disease activity. It is not uncommon for pregnant women to experience a worsening of morning stiffness and back pain during pregnancy. Up to 60% of women may suffer a flare of disease activity during the six months following delivery. Pregnancy complications attributable to AS are rare; the complication rates for babies born to mothers with AS are similar to those expected in the population of mothers without AS.

Women with AS should not take nonsteroidal anti-inflammatory drugs (NSAIDs) during pregnancy. Similarly, women who plan to breastfeed should not take NSAIDs. During pregnancy, inflammation may be treated with acetaminophen (Tylenol) or corticosteroid injections. However, prior to taking any medications during pregnancy, you should consult your obstetrician and your rheumatologist.

Question: Will sexual activity become a problem now that I've been diagnosed with AS?

Answer: When you're in pain or feeling tired—not uncommon symptoms of AS—having sexual relations may not be at the top of your "To Do" list. However, there is no evidence that sexual relations are affected by having AS, other than using good common sense that dictates one should avoid any physical activity that causes pain. The good news is that when you are feeling stimulated, sexual activity may be therapeutic, resulting in the release of chemicals known as endorphins that alleviate stress and relieve pain.

Question: My AS is fairly well controlled. However, I've heard people talk about my getting additional help from complementary treatments. Are there nontraditional treatments that might help a condition like mine?

Answer: Nonsteroidal anti-inflammatory drugs, anti-TNF inhibitors, and steroid injections are the primary traditional treatments for AS. Patients seeking nontraditional therapy may be motivated to do so as a result of a poor response to these traditional medications. Complementary and alternative medicine (CAM) is defined by the National Institutes of Health as "a group of diverse medical and health care systems, practices, and products that are not presently considered to be a part of conventional medicine."

At the present time, there is no rigorous scientific evidence to suggest that patients with AS can benefit from the use of CAM. There are, however, patient reports that CAM helps alleviate the symptoms of AS. Acupuncture, massage, yoga therapy, tai chi, and the use of a TENS (transcutaneous electrical nerve stimulation) unit may be helpful. There is very little information about the benefits of Chinese herbal medications; given that these medications are unregulated by the Food and Drug Administration, caution is advised. Use of any nontraditional treatments should be discussed first with your rheumatologist. Chiropractic treatments that involve spinal manipulation are not recommended for patients with AS because of the possibility of injury.

GLOSSARY

Acute anterior uveitis (AAU). An inflammation of the iris and ciliary body that occurs in the front part of the eye. Also referred to as *uveitis*.

Aortic regurgitation. A condition that occurs when the aortic value of the heart weakens and prevents the valve from closing tightly. Blood then flows backwards and this process can damage the heart.

Articular process. Articular processes are extensions outwards from the vertebral bodies and form the joints of the spine, and vary in form based on location in the spine.

ARTS-1. A recently discovered gene that may play a role in the development of ankylosing spondylitis.

Asymptomatic. A disease is asymptomatic if a patient is a carrier for the disease but experiences no symptoms.

Axial skeleton. The axial skeleton consists of 80 bones in the head and trunk of the body, and is divided into five parts: skull, ossicles of the inner ear, hyoid bone of the throat, rib cage, and the vertebral column.

Bisphosphonates. A class of drugs that bind to bone surfaces and prevent the loss of bone mass.

Calcification. A condition that occurs when calcium salts build up in soft tissue, causing the soft tissue to harden.

Cartilage. A type of connective tissue found throughout the body, including at the joints and between bones in the spine. Cartilage is stiff and inflexible.

Cauda equina. Nerve roots at the end of the spinal cord form a structure known as the *cauda equina*, or "horse's tail." These nerves provide innervation to the lower trunk, legs, bowels, bladder, and sexual organs.

Cervical curve. One of several spinal curves that support the body. The cervical curve is the first curve to develop, a process that occurs when a baby learns to lift its head.

Cervical vertebrae. The first seven vertebrae located at the top of the spinal column. Collectively, these vertebrae comprise the cervical vertebrae. The cervical vertebrae provide the flexible framework for the neck, as well as support for the head.

Cervicothoracic. The cervicothoracic area encompasses the neck and the region between the head and the abdomen.

Chlamydia trachomatis. A type of bacteria belonging to the genus *Chlamydia.*

Coccyx. Commonly referred to as the "tailbone," the coccyx is located at the bottom of the spinal column and is the final segment of the vertebral column.

Conduction system disturbances. Abnormalities in the conduction pathways of the heart.

Conjunctivitis. Swelling or infection of the lining of the eyelids and outside surfaces of the eye.

Cortex. The hard outer layer of bones.

C-reactive protein (CRP). C-reactive protein is a type of protein in the blood that rises in response to inflammation. C-reactive protein tests are used as one measure of inflammation.

Crohn's disease. A type of inflammatory bowel disease.

Cytokine. A type of small protein secreted by cells within the immune system.

Dactylitis. A condition in which entire fingers or toes are very swollen and look like sausages.

Decompression surgery. Decompression surgery is a general term that refers to any surgery that involves taking the pressure off the spinal cord or nerves to restore neurologic function or prevent neurologic dysfunction.

Diffuse idiopathic skeletal hyperostosis (DISH). A type of degenerative arthritis characterized by a calcification or a bony hardening of ligaments at the point of attachment to the spine.

Enteropathy. Any disorder of the intestine.

Enteropathic arthritis. Enteropathic arthritis is associated with inflammatory bowel disease and is a type of arthritis that involves the lower peripheral joints, such as knees, ankles, or feet.

Entheses. The site at which a tendon, ligament, or muscle inserts into bone.

Enthesitis. Inflammation of the entheses.

ERAP1. Endoplasmic reticulum aminopeptidase 1; a gene associated with ankylosing spondylitis.

Erythrocyte sedimentation rate (ESR). A measure of inflammation.

Facet joints. Joints that join the bones of the spine together and enable the body to move, twist, and bend.

Foramen magnum. A hole in the base of the skull through which the spinal cord leaves the brain.

Gastrointestinal tract. The part of the body that extends from the mouth to the anus and encompasses the stomach and intestines.

Genitourinary tract. The system of organs that includes the reproductive organs and urinary system.

HLA-B27. Human leukocyte antigen; a type of antigen (molecule) strongly associated with ankylosing spondylitis.

IL-23R. Interleukin-23 receptor; a gene associated with ankylosing spondylitis.

Inflammation. A response of body tissues to injury or irritation; characterized by pain and swelling and redness and heat.

Inflammatory bowel disease (IBD). A term used to describe two chronic diseases that cause inflammation of the intestines: ulcerative colitis and Crohn's disease.

Intervertebral discs. In between each of the vertebra that forms the vertebral column are intervertebral discs. These discs are comprised of a fibrous cartilage that acts as a shock absorber and allows the back to move.

Iritis. Inflammation of the iris; also known as acute anterior uveitis.

Lamina. The top part of the spinal canal that covers the spinal cord and its nerves on which there are two to three types of bony extensions called *processes*.

Left ventricular dysfunction. A heart condition in which the left ventricle of the heart does not function properly.

Ligaments. A type of fibrous tissue that connects bones to other bones.

Lumbar curve. The portion of the spine that begins in the middle of the last thoracic vertebra and ends at the sacrovertebral angle. The lumber curve develops as the child begins to walk.

Lumbar lordosis. An exaggerated inward curvature of the lower back region.

Lumbar vertebrae. One of five spinal regions, the lumbar vertebrae are the largest bones in the spinal column. These bones are attached to many of the back muscles, and function to support the body's weight.

Magnetic resonance imaging (MRI). A noninvasive diagnostic imaging test that uses an electromagnetic process to allow for the visualization of the detailed internal structure of the body.

Marrow. Flexible tissue located in the hollow interior of bones.

Modified Stoke ankylosing spondylitis score. A method of scoring radiographic damage in ankylosing spondylitis.

Musculoskeletal system. The muscles, bones, joints and related structures of the body.

Neurologic. Pertaining to the nervous system.

Nonsteroidal anti-inflammatory drug (NSAID). A type of drug treatment used to reduce inflammation in patients with ankylosing spondylitis.

Occiput-to-wall distance. A measure of spinal mobility that measures the distance someone's head is tilted forward.

Osteoporosis. Thinning of the bones.

Osteotomy. A type of spine surgery used to correct spinal deformities by cutting and realigning the bone.

Paleopathology. The study of diseases in ancient times through analyses of skeletal and other body part remains.

Pedicles. Part of the spinal canal, pedicles attach the lamina to the vertebral body.

Pelvic curve. The portion of the spine that begins at the sacrovertebral articulation and ends at the point of the coccyx. The pelvic curve is also known as the sacral curve.

Peripheral arthritis. A type of arthritis that primarily targets the peripheral limbs (arms and legs) as opposed to arthritis of the spine.

Psoriasis. A skin condition in which dead skin cells build up to form thick, dry scaly patches on the elbows, knees, scalp, or lower spine. Fingernails may become pitted, discolored, and pieces may fall from the nail beds.

Peripheral joint synovitis. An inflammation of the synovial tissue lined joints that occurs in about 50% of ankylosing spondylitis patients, targeting the hips, knees, ankles, fingers and toes.

Prevalence. A term used by epidemiologists to refer to the total number of cases of a disease in a given population at a specific time.

Pulmonary. Pertaining to the lungs.

Reactive arthritis (ReA). A type of arthritis that occurs in reaction to a triggering event such as a bacterial infection. Reactive arthritis usually occurs from infections either the gastrointestinal or urinary tract. There is some speculation that reactive arthritis may also occur coincident with the human immunodeficiency virus (HIV).

Sacral curve. The portion of the spine that begins at the sacrovertebral articulation, and ends at the point of the coccyx. The sacral curve is also known as the pelvic curve.

Sacroiliitis. An inflammation of the sacroiliac joints. The sacroiliac joints connect the lower spine and the pelvis.

Sacrum. A triangular shaped bone located just below the lumbar vertebrae.

Salmonella. A type of severe food poisoning.

Secondary amyloidosis. The buildup of amyloid (a type of protein) in body organs or tissue that is related, or secondary, to chronic inflammatory disease.

Spinal canal. The spinal canal includes the vertebral body, pedicles, lamina and, in the lower back region, the nerve roots of the lower spine. The canal refers to the opening where the spinal cord and nerves are located.

Spinal column. The spinal column is composed of an intricate and complex group of muscles, ligaments, bones, and tendons that support the body, hold it upright, and allow it to twist and bend. The spinal column is also referred to as backbone, spine, or vertebral column.

Spinal cord. A long, thin, tubular group of tissue and cells that extends from the brain to the space between the first and second lumbar vertebrae.

Spinal fusion. A type of spine surgery that fuses two or more vertebrae.

Spinal instrumentation. Used after spinal fusion surgery, spinal instrumentation uses hooks, rods, and wires to redistribute stress on the bones and keep them properly aligned during the healing process.

Spine kyphosis. An exaggerated curve in the lower back. Spine kyphosis is also referred to as "hunchback."

Spinous process. A bony protrusion that points straight back toward the skin behind the spine. These protrusions can be felt as bumps on the back of the upper body.

Spondyloarthropathies (SPAs). A group of inflammatory rheumatologic diseases characterized by an inflammation of the axial skeleton, entheses (bony insertions of ligaments and tendons), and peripheral joints. Other systems such as the eyes, skin, gut, and genitourinary tract may be affected as well.

Subluxation. This term refers to the situation when one or more of the bones in the spine moves out of position, creating pressure or irritation on the spinal nerves.

Syndesmophytes. A bony growth seen in the ligaments of the spine.

Synovitis. An inflammation of the synovial joints.

Systemic. Affecting the entire system.

Tendon. Connective tissue made of collagen that connects muscle to bone.

Tenosynovitis. An inflammation of the fluid-filled sheath surrounding a tendon.

Thoracic curve. Curve corresponding to the thoracic region of the spine.

Thoracic vertebrae. Bones that form the rear anchor of the rib cage. The thoracic vertebrae form a transition between the cervical vertebrae above and the lumbar vertebrae below.

Thoracolumbar junction. Section of the vertebral column beginning at the eleventh thoracic vertebra and ending at the first lumbar vertebra.

Transverse process. A set of laminar extensions that vary in shape and form depending upon location in the spine. The transverse processes point out to the sides.

Tumor necrosis factor-alpha (TNF-α) inhibitor. A class of therapeutics known as *biologics* that work to block the inflammatory response evoked by a type of cytokine known as *tumor necrosis factor*.

Ulcerative colitis (UC). A type of inflammatory bowel disease.

Uveitis. An inflammation of the iris and ciliary body that occurs in the front part of the eye. Also referred to as *acute anterior uveitis*.

Vertebrae. The collection of bones that comprise the spinal column. The vertebrae of the spinal column are grouped into five regions and the vertebral bodies increase in size moving from the top of the spinal column to the bottom.

Yersinia. A Gram-negative bacteria.

INDEX

Note: Page references followed by "*f*" and "*t*" denote figures and tables, respectively.

Acetaminophen (Tylenol), 107
Acupuncture, 108
Acute anterior uveitis (AAU),
     35, 58, 67
Adalimumab (Humira), 78
     for psoriatic arthritis, 62
Age, and AS incidence, 15
Amenhotep II, 11
Amyloid, 39
Amyloidosis, 39–40
Analgesics, and kidney
     problems, 40
Ankylosis. *See* Bone ankylosis;
     Spinal ankylosis
Ankylosing Spondylitis
     International Federation, 72
Anthraxin receptor 2 (ANTXR2)
     gene, 99
Antibiotics, for reactive arthritis, 60
Anti-TNF therapy, 100, 101, 106
     for juvenile-onset ankylosing
     spondylitis (JOAS), 54
Aortic regurgitation, 38
Arthritis, 30
     enteropathic arthritis, 63–64

peripheral arthritis, 64
psoriatic arthritis, 60–63
reactive arthritis, 57, 58–60
rheumatoid arthritis, 30
spondyloarthritis, definition, 57.
     See also Spondyloarthritis
     (SpA)
Articular processes, 22, 23*f*
ARTS-1 gene, 16
Assessment of SpondyloArthritis
     international Society
     (ASAS), 9
Automobile safety, 92–93
Axial skeleton, 5, 5*f*, 57

Backbone. *See* Spine
Back pain, low. *See* Chronic
     inflammatory low
     back pain
Back stretch exercise, 73*f*, 74
Bechterew, Vladimir, 13
Biologics, 36, 48, 54, 60, 63, 66, 67.
     See also Tumor necrosis
     factor-alpha (TNF-α)
     inhibitors

Bisphosphonates, 77
  for osteoporosis, 47–48, 77
Blood test, 32, 57
Bone ankylosis, 100
Bone density preservation, 47
Bone formation, new, 5, 45, 62,
    98, 101
Bone health, 45–48. *See also*
    Osteoporosis
  fractures and, 46–47
  treatment, for osteoporosis,
    47–48
Brodie, Benjamin, 12

Calcium, for osteoporosis, 47
Cardiovascular system, and AS,
    37–38
Cauda equina, 22
Cauda equina syndrome, 41–42
Cervical curve, 20–21
Cervical vertebrae, 18, 19*f*, 20*f*
Chest wall rigidity, 39
Children
  ankylosing spondylitis in. *See*
    Juvenile-onset ankylosing
    spondylitis (JOAS)
  effect of AS on caring for, 92
  spondyloarthritis in.
    See Juvenile-onset
    spondyloarthritis
Chlamydia trachomatis, 59
Chronic inflammatory low back
    pain, 27–28
  characteristics of, 28
  Classification criteria
    for AS, 7–9, 8*t*
    for psoriatic arthritis, 61–62
Clinical presentation, of AS, 27–31
  arthritis, 30
  chronic inflammatory low back
    pain, 27–28
  enthesitis, 29

osteoporosis, 30–31
Coccyx, 18, 19, 19*f*, 20*f*
Colombo, Realdo, 12
Complementary and alternative
    medicine (CAM), 108–9
  definition of, 108
Complete heart block, 38
Conduction system disturbances,
    37, 38
Connor, Bernard, 12
Controlled stretch exercise, 88–89
Corticosteroids, 76–77
  for enteropathic arthritis, 64
  for JOAS, 54
  for peripheral arthritis, 64
  during pregnancy, 107
Cosimo il Veccho, 12
C-reactive protein (CRP), 32
Crohn's disease (CD), 16, 42, 63–64
  symptoms of, 63

Dactylitis, 61, 62*f*, 67
Daily activity. *See* Physical/daily
    activity
Decompression surgery, 81, 82
Deep breathing exercise, 88, 89
Diagnosis, of AS, 7–9, 14, 31–33, 98
Diffuse idiopathic skeletal
    hyperostosis (DISH), 11
Disease-modifying anti-rheumatic
    drugs (DMARDs), 77–78
  for psoriatic arthritis, 62
  for reactive arthritis, 60
Disease process, of AS, 5, 7*f*
Doctor, communication with, 103–4
Driving, automobile safety, 92–93

Education, patient, 71, 72
Effects, of AS, 5–6
Endoplasmic reticulum
    aminopeptidase 1
    (ERAP1) gene, 99

Enteropathic arthritis, 63–64
  symptoms, 64
  treatment, 64
Enteropathy, definition of, 63
Enthesitis, 29, 29*f*, 51–52
Erectile dysfunction, 40
Erythrocyte sedimentation rate
  (ESR), 32
Etanercept (Enbrel), 78
  for psoriatic arthritis, 62
Ethnicity, and AS incidence, 15
  and HLA-B27 prevalence, 32
Etymology, of AS, 11
Exercises, 73–74, 73*f*, 88–89. *See
  also* Physical/daily activity
  for JOAS, 54
Extensor muscles, 23
Eye. *See also* Ophthalmologic
  system, and AS
  anatomy of, 36*f*
  inflammation, 106. *See also* Acute
  anterior uveitis (AAU)

Facet joints, 21, 21*f*
Fatigue, 91
Flexor muscles, 23
Florentine Medici family, skeletal
  remains studies, 12
Foramen magnum, 21
Fractures, 46–47. *See also*
  Osteoporosis
  diagnosis of, 46–47
  risk factors, 46
  spinal, 40–41
  stress, 41
  vertebral, 41, 46–47
Future prospects for diagnosis and
  treatment of AS, 97–102

Gastrointestinal system, and AS,
  42–43
Gender, and AS incidence, 15

Genetics, 16, 98–99. *See also*
  Inheritance
Genitourinary tract. *See*
  Reproductive system, and
  AS; Urinary system, and AS
Golimumab (Simponi), 78
  for psoriatic arthritis, 62
Guiliano Duco de Nemours, 12
Gut. *See* Gastrointestinal system,
  and AS

Handicap parking places, 93
Heart. *See also* Cardiovascular
  system, and AS
  anatomy of, 37*f*
  valve dysfunction, 37, 38
Heredity. *See* Genetics; Inheritance
Hip disease, 30
Hippocrates, 11
Hip replacement surgery, 83, 83*f*
History, of AS, 11–14
  paleopathology, 11
HLA-B27 gene, 14, 16, 32, 37, 51,
  57, 59, 65, 97, 98–99, 107
Horse's tail. *See Cauda equina*
Hunchback, 28

Ibuprofen (Advil, Motrin), 75
Infections, of artificial joints, 84
Inflammation, and disease activity,
  98, 100–1
Inflammatory back pain. *See*
  Chronic inflammatory low
  back pain
Inflammatory bowel disease (IBD),
  42–43, 63–64, 67, 98,
  101–2
  treatment, 64
Infliximab (Remicade), 78
  for psoriatic arthritis, 62
Inheritance of AS, 107. *See also*
  Genetics

Interleukin-1 receptor 2 (IL1R2) gene, 99
Interleukin-23 receptor (IL-23R) gene, 16, 99
Intervertebral discs, 19–20
Iritis, 12, 35
Irritation of spinal nerves, 41

Joint replacement surgery, 81, 82–84
Juvenile-onset ankylosing spondylitis (JOAS), 51–55
 clinical presentation, 51–52
 diagnosis and treatment, 53–55
 symptoms, 52–53
Juvenile-onset spondyloarthritis, 65–66
 symptoms, 65

Kidney. *See* Renal system, and AS
Knee replacement surgery, 83, 84*f*
 arthroplasty, 84*f*

Lamina, 22
Left ventricular dysfunction, 37, 38
Lorenzo il Magnifico, 12
Lumbar lordosis, 28
Lumbar vertebrae, 18, 19, 22, 19*f*, 20*f*
Lumbar curve, 20
Lungs. *See* Pulmonary system, and AS

Magnetic resonance imaging (MRI), 14, 32–33
Management of AS, 71–79
 nonpharmacologic treatment, 72–74
 exercise and physical therapy, 73–74
 patient education, 72

pharmacologic treatment, 74–79
 bisphosphonates, 77
 corticosteroids, 76–77
 disease-modifying anti-rheumatic drugs, 77–78
 nonsteroidal anti-inflammatory drugs, 74–76
 tumor necrosis factor-alpha inhibitors, 78–79
Marie, Pierre, 13
Massage, 108
Medical history, 31, 32
 and JOAS, 53, 54
Medications, disclosing information about, 105
Merneptah, 11
Methotrexate
 for psoriatic arthritis, 62
 for reactive arthritis, 60
 for rheumatoid arthritis, 77–78
Modified New York 1984 classification criteria, 7, 8*t*
Morbus Strumpell-Marie-Bechterew, 13

Naproxen (Aleve, Naprosyn), 75
Nerves. *See* Neurologic system, and AS
Neurologic system, and AS, 40–42
Nonsteroidal anti-inflammatory drugs (NSAIDs), 74–76, 97, 100
 adverse effects, 75–76
 for enteropathic arthritis, 64
 for JOAS, 54
 and kidney problems, 40
 for psoriatic arthritis, 62
 in pregnancy, 107
 for reactive arthritis, 60

Nurse, role in JOAS, 54
Nutritionist, role in JOAS, 54

Oblique muscles, 23
Occupational therapy, for psoriatic
    arthritis, 63
Ophthalmologic system, and AS,
    35–36
Ophthalmologist
    for treatment of JOAS, 54
    for treatment of uveitis, 36
Osteoporosis, 30–31, 45
    treatment for, 47–48
Osteotomy, 81–82

Pacemaker, 38
Pelvic curve. *See* Sacral curve
Peripheral arthritis, 64, 67, 78
Peripheral joint synovitis, 30
Physical/daily activity, 87–94
    automobile safety, 92–93
    child care, 92
    controlled stretch exercise, 88–89
    deep breathing exercise, 89
    and fatigue, 91
    posture, 94
    recreational activities, 91–92
    smoking cessation, 93
    workplace activity, 90–91
Physical examination, 31–32
Physical therapist, for treatment of
    JOAS, 54
Physical therapy, 71, 73, 74
    for JOAS, 54
    for psoriatic arthritis, 63
Piero il Gottoso, 12
Posture, 73, 94
    and JOAS, 52, 54
Pregnancy, and AS, 107
    Prevalence, of AS, 15
Processes, bony extensions,
    22, 23*f*, 28

Proteinuria, 40
Psoriasis, definition of, 60
Psoriatic arthritis, 60–63
    characteristics, 61
    classification criteria, 61–62
    onset of, 61
    treatment, 62–63
Psychologist
    for juvenile-onset ankylosing
        spondylitis, 54
    for juvenile-onset
        spondyloarthritis, 66
Pulmonary system, and AS, 39

Radiologic examination, 32
Ramses the Great, 11, 12
Reactive arthritis (ReA), 57, 58–60
    duration of, 59
    symptoms, 58–59
    treatment of, 60
Recreational activities, 91–92
Reiter's syndrome, 12
Renal system, and AS, 35, 39–40
Reproductive system, and
        AS, 40
Restricted chest capacity, surgical
        challenges of, 85
Rheumatoid arthritis (RA), 30
    and spondyloarthritis, 57
Rheumatoid variants, 57
Roentgen, Wilhelm, 14

Sachs, Bernard, 13
Sacral curve, 20
Sacrum, 18, 19
Salmonella, 59
Secondary amyloidosis, 39–40
Seronegative spondyloarthritis, 57
Sexual activity, 59, 108
Sexual dysfunction, 40
Shigella, 59
Smoking cessation, 93, 105–6

Spine, 17–23
  axial spine, 6*f*
  canal, 22
  curves of, 20–21
  flattening of the lumbar spine, 28
  fractures, 40–41, 46
  fused, 13*f*
  inflammation, factors associated
    with, 99–100
  instrumentation and fusion, 82
  irritation of spinal nerves, 41
  osteoporosis, 45. *See also*
    Osteoporosis
  rate of progression of spinal
    ankylosis, 98
  spinal arthritis, 97
  structure and function of, 17–23
  surgery, 81–82
Spinous process, 22, 23*f*
Spondylitis Association of
    America, 72, 88
Spondyloarthritis (SpA), 57–67
  enteropathic arthritis, 63–64
  juvenile-onset spondyloarthritis,
    65–66
  psoriatic arthritis, 60–63
  reactive arthritis, 58–60
  undifferentiated
    spondyloarthritis, 66–67
Spondyloarthropathies (SPAs), 5
Standing. *See* Controlled stretch
    exercise
Steroid medication, for AAU, 36
Stress fractures, 41
Strumpell, A., 12–13
Subluxation, 41
Sulfasalazine
  for psoriatic arthritis, 62
  for rheumatoid arthritis, 77–78
Surgery, for AS, 81–85
  challenges, 85
  joint replacement surgery, 82–84

  spine surgery, 81–82
Synovial joints, 21, 30

Tai chi, 88, 109
Tail bone. *See* Coccyx
Tensosynovitis, 61
Thoracic vertebrae, 18–19, 19*f*, 20*f*
Thoracic curve, 20
Transcutaneous electrical nerve
    stimulation (TENS), 109
Transverse processes, 22, 23*f*
Tumor necrosis factor (TNF) α
    inhibitors, 78–79, 97
  adverse effects, 79
  for enteropathic arthritis, 64
  for psoriatic arthritis, 62

Ulcerative colitis (UC), 42, 63–64
  symptoms, 63
Undifferentiated spondyloarthritis
    (uSpA), 66–67
  symptoms, 67
Urinary system, and AS, 40
Uveitis, 100, 106. *See also* Acute
    anterior uveitis (AAU)
  and JOAS, 53, 55

Valve replacement surgery, for
    aortic regurgitation, 38
Vertebrae, 5, 11, 18–19, 19*f*, 20*f*,
    22. *See also* Spine
  fractures, 41, 46–47
Vertebral column. *See* Spine
Vitamin D, for osteoporosis, 47

Workplace activity, 90–91

X-rays, 7, 8, 12, 14, 32, 33, 47

Yersinia, 59
Yoga therapy, 88, 109